TEND TO YOUR SPIRIT

MINDFUL LIVING WITH CHRONIC ILLNESS

JULIANNE LEPP AND FLORENCE CAPLOW

Boston
Skinner House Books

www.skinnerhouse.org

Printed in the United States

Cover design by Alex Camlin
Text design by Tim Holtz
Illustrations by Alyssa Alarcón Santo

print ISBN: 978-1-55896-969-8
eBook ISBN: 978-1-55896-970-4

6 5 4 3 2 1
29 28 27 26 25

Cataloging-in-Publication information on file with the Library of Congress

We gratefully acknowledge the following permissions:

"All That Is Glorious Around Us" from *Radiance: Poems* by Barbara Crooker, © 2005. barbaracrooker.com.

"Badass Warriors Among Us" by Tandi Rogers.

"bare bones" by Ullie-Kaye. etsy.com/shop/UllieKayePoetry.

"Camas Lilies" by Lynn Unger. Lynnungar.com.

"Don't Know Mind" by Zen Master Bon Soeng. Originally published on emptygatezen.com.

Excerpt from "French Chocolates" from *Like a Beggar* by Ellen Bass, © 2014. Reprinted with permission of the Permissions Company, LLC, on behalf of Copper Canyon Press. Coppercanyonpress.org.

Excerpts from *Beyond the Mailbox: A Life with Chronic Illness* by Pat Gavula, © 2023.

Darlene Cohen, excerpts from *Turning Suffering Inside Out: A Zen Approach to Living with Physical and Emotional Pain.* Copyright © 2000 by Darlene Cohen. Reprinted by arrangement with The Permissions Company, LLC on behalf of Shambhala Publications Inc., Boulder, Colorado, shambhala.com.

"Having it Together" by Sarah York from *Into the Wilderness.* Apollo Ranch Press, 2000.

"The Map You Make Yourself" © Jan Richardson from *Circle of Grace: A Book of Blessings for the Seasons.* janrichardson.com.

"Light De Light" by Peter Levitt. peterlevitt.com.

"Spell for Rest and Renewal" by Atena O. Danner. atenadannercreative.com.

"Take Courage, Friends" by Wayne Arnason.

"To Know the Dark" from *New Collected Poems* by Wendell Berry, © 1970. Reprinted with the permission of The Permissions Company, LLC, on behalf of Counterpoint Press. counterpointpress.com.

Toni Bernhard, excerpts from *How to Live Well with Chronic Pain and Illness: A Mindful Guide.* Copyright © 2015 by Toni Bernhard. Reprinted with the permission of The Permissions Company, LLC on behalf of Wisdom Publications, wisdompubs.org.

Contents

SUMMER

Introduction

*One day you will tell the story of what you
are going through now and it will become
part of someone else's survival guide.*

Brené Brown

If you have picked up this book, you are most likely someone who is
living with chronic illness or pain. Perhaps you are newly diagnosed
and still reeling with what this may mean for you; perhaps your condition has affected you for many years and you are looking for new
ways of living with what you have; or perhaps you are seeing physical
improvements but find that your spirit is still not healed. Or perhaps
you are in a caregiving role or are thinking of giving this book to someone you know who is facing the challenges of illness or pain.

Whatever your circumstances, you have probably found that there
are many difficult emotions associated with chronic physical challenges: grief, despair, frustration, shame, and a host of others. These

emotions can be as hard or harder to live with than the chronic condition itself. There are also, of course, moments of comfort, peace, hope, connection, and presence, and these are important too.

We wrote *Tend to Your Spirit* because we both live with a chronic, painful, and sometimes disabling illness (rheumatoid arthritis, or RA), and we are both Unitarian Universalist ministers. We want to offer you what we have learned about living with chronic illness, spiritual practices that we have used and taught that can bring some ease, and words and images that inspire our spirits from day to day.

In this book you will find stories from our lives, stories from others whose life circumstances and illnesses are different from ours— many from marginalized and silenced communities—meditations, journal prompts, quotes, poetry, and music. This book is meant to be contemplatively browsed and savored. It is meant to be an encouraging, thought-provoking spiritual companion through the seasons of chronic illness, a companion we wish we had had ourselves.

We also envision *Tend to Your Spirit* as a study guide for small groups, which we are calling Seasons Circles. Read the chapter "Using This Book in Small Groups" in the back of the book to learn more.

The Stages and Seasons of a Chronic Condition

Some people talk about the stages of learning to live with a chronic illness or injury. Joy Selak and Dr. Steven Overman, in the book *You Don't Look Sick! Living Well with Invisible Chronic Illness*, describe these stages this way, based on the work of Patricia Fennell:

1. Crisis/Getting Sick includes the shock, anger, fear, and loss experienced when a person first gets sick or injured or is first diagnosed with a chronic disease.

2. Stabilization/Being Sick, where there is more acceptance of having a chronic condition and the person begins to work with their circumstances more actively.

3. Resolution, the third phase, is a deeper part of Being Sick, where there is room for grieving the old life that has been lost or changed and accepting that the illness or injury is not short term. (Though that doesn't mean you're not still working to be as healthy as possible!)

4. And finally, Integration/Living Well, when a person finds value, meaning, and purpose in their life as it is, no matter how sick or healthy the body may be.

The reality is that if an illness or injury lasts more than a few months, this cycle will probably recur again and again and will begin again with a new diagnosis.

As we were considering the structure of this book, we decided to use the metaphors of the four seasons to represent these four stages and the cycle as a whole: fall for crisis, winter for stabilization, spring for resolution, and summer for integration. Within each season, there are four chapters devoted to some of the challenges you may experience there and ways to live well, wherever you are in your journey.

We hope that this book can help you move from surviving your condition to thriving in your circumstances in every season. As Darlene Cohen, author of *Turning Suffering Inside Out*: *A Zen Approach to Living with Physical and Emotional Pain*, wrote:

> The world that opened to me through engaging the physical suffering and mental anguish caused by my disease has turned out to be inexpressibly rich. Because if we can engage with our

suffering—connect with it, dance with it, tease it, coax it, curse it, as well as trying to change it, just consider it our lives, experience it as our lives, the only lives we have—it changes the quality of that suffering. It's not just our suffering; it's everything.

This is what we hope for you.

Tools We Offer

For each season, you will find an introductory essay followed by four chapters on distinct themes. Although each theme is different, there will be some common elements.

- Contemplative reflections by the authors on that theme

- Thematic spiritual practices

- Journal prompts

- Sticky note reminders that might inspire you to create your own notes

- Reflection questions, which can be used on your own or in a group

- "Gold leaves" (our version of gold stars) where you can celebrate ways you are doing well

- Quotes and poetry for insight and enjoyment

- For some themes, stories from individuals with diverse identities that explore their experience with chronic illness or pain and offer advice and wisdom

- A curated playlist of music on the theme. These links are also available on our companion website, tend-to-your-spirit.info.

At the back of the book, you will find guided meditations for each season. These guided meditations are also available on our companion website. You will also find further resources and reading for your journey and a guide for Seasons Circles, small study groups working with the practices in this book.

Suggestions for How to Use This Book

Because this book is meant to be a balm for your spirit, rather than another item on your long to-do list, we invite you to use it in whatever ways are most helpful for you, with an attitude of gentleness toward yourself. It is meant to be savored, to be nibbled upon, rather than read from beginning to end. You can start in the beginning, or you can start in the season or feeling that feels most true for you right now.

If you are a journal keeper, perhaps the journal prompts will lead you into new territory. You can also use the questions to go deeper in journaling, or, if you are part of a support group, you may want to use the questions as a guide for discussion in the group.

If you are a meditator or an aspiring meditator, you can have someone read the guided meditations to you or use the companion website to listen to the meditations. Or perhaps you want to take up one of the spiritual practices for a day or a week or longer.

Maybe a quote strikes you in just the right way. If so, you can copy it out and put it on your fridge or your mirror. Or maybe, on a day that you feel discouraged, you can give yourself a gold leaf or rock out to one of the playlists.

The readings are intentionally short because often our attention spans are limited when we are in pain or experiencing fatigue. There is no wrong way to read or use this book!

Who We Are

We are both Unitarian Universalist ministers. We are white, cisgender, queer women in mid-life, and we are both diagnosed with active rheumatoid arthritis.

Julianne was diagnosed with rheumatoid arthritis in 2021 and has been learning about living with chronic illness as a mother, partner, and full-time minister. She previously worked as a professional massage therapist and reiki practitioner with a focus on clients struggling with grief and addiction. Since 2010, Julianne has served as the solo minister of the Unitarian Universalist Congregation in Eau Claire, Wisconsin, and she obtained her certification in Spiritual Direction through Meadville Lombard Theological School in 2025. Julianne is a published poet and game designer and a long-time explorer of labyrinths, spiritual practice, and earth-centered spirituality. She lives in Wisconsin with her spouse Karl, children Ehren and Kendra, mother-in-law Eleta, and four beloved cats.

Florence has been affected by chronic autoimmune illnesses of various sorts since 1999. For the first three years of being ill, she did not have a diagnosis. Fatigue, pain, and an unreliable body have been her companions for more than two decades. She was diagnosed with another autoimmune disease, rheumatoid arthritis, in 2021. She served Unitarian Universalist congregations in Washington, Colorado, and Illinois before leaving full-time ministry due to increased illness. She is also a Zen Buddhist priest and teacher, teaching through Cloud Way Zen, and a change coach and spiritual director. She lives in Central Illinois with two pandemic cats, a vibrant garden, and kind neighbors for company.

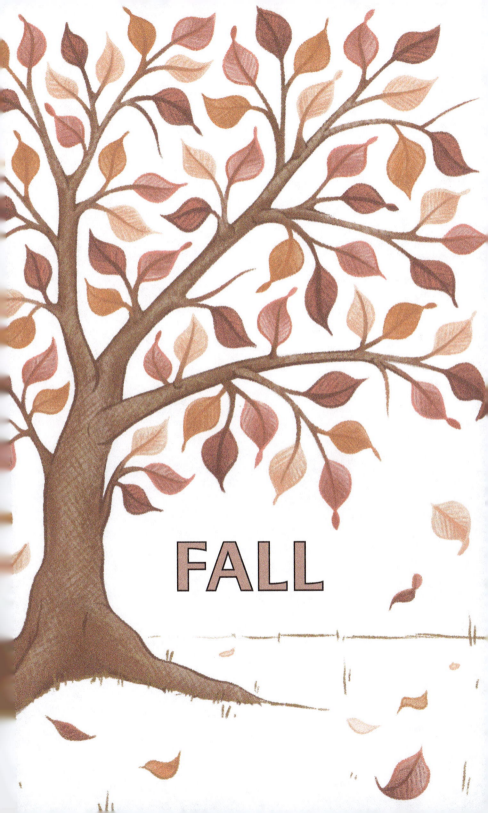

FALL

By Julianne Lepp

Tessa Miller writes in *What Doesn't Kill You: A Life with Chronic Illness—Lessons from a Body in Revolt,* "I became a professional patient, and a good one. I learned that bodies can be inexplicably resilient and curiously fragile. I would never get better, and that would change *everything*: the way I think about my body, my health, my relationships, my work, and my life. When things get rough, people like to say, "this too shall pass." But what happens when 'this' never goes away?"

It can be devastating to get a diagnosis, knowing that your life will never be the same. I was so angry when my rheumatologist told me I'd have to take major medications for the rest of my life to counter the crippling effects of rheumatoid arthritis. I was unprepared for the quick changes in my health and stamina. Resisting the need for rest, I'd push through until I just couldn't do anymore, and then I felt defeated and frustrated when I had to ask for help or couldn't do what I used to be able to do.

Autumn heralds breakdown, decay, and a reduction of life to the basic elements. All life returns to the earth, dies away, and new life emerges again. In the topsy-turvy, often unpredictable world of chronic illness, seasons and cycles can offer comfort and stability, like the rising and setting of the sun. Autumn's cooler winds whisper of the beauty of letting go and making room for new things.

With any change, and particularly a new diagnosis, rage may rise up when least expected at the unfairness of pain and limitation. There may be grief at the loss that chronic illness brings. Beauty and loss, transformation and change end up all mixed together. What are the lessons in what is dying away? Fall can be a time for release and reflection. A new chronic illness or condition can be like this too, when we are forced to evaluate what to keep and what to let go, and how to use our energy and time.

When I was first diagnosed with rheumatoid arthritis, I had so much inflammation that I couldn't lift items over five pounds, I couldn't use something as basic as scissors, and it was extremely painful to type. My feet were so swollen I was unable to stand for long periods or walk without pain. Chronic illness can mean we may no longer be able to do the tasks that we once did or that we can't approach our lives, careers, and pastimes in the same way. Maybe we must move more slowly and carefully or need more assistance than we did before. We may be faced with sudden changes in health and ability, whereas others are so gradual that they might not be noticed until it takes us by surprise. Sometimes we have to stop doing hobbies we once loved because of hands that can no longer knit, feet that won't support running, or eyesight or brain fog that prevents driving alone.

The challenge with these losses is to acknowledge and notice them, just as we can notice how the leaves fall and bring new nourishment to the earth. Each challenge, each struggle is a resource or experience to draw from. When we can notice the toll of pain or the gifts of acknowledging a limitation, that is fuel for living more intentionally. Examination rather than avoidance, integration rather than hiding from these incredibly hard experiences, can lead to transformation.

Autumn gives us permission to pause and notice the changes happening right now or reflect on what has already changed. As we move from warmer seasons toward the colder, more reflective time of year, it is the signal to start slowing down and drawing our intentions inward. Fall can give us a time to tap into feelings that we might shove down in busy lives or to cope with pain—feelings of anger, grief, invisibility, or shame. There can be anger when people disbelieve our illnesses and conditions, such as doctors that don't take us seriously or friends and coworkers that minimize our experience of pain and illness. We may struggle with spending months or years hoping for diagnosis, relief, or medicine. We may feel despair when our conditions are dismissed because they are not easily observed. And we may feel invisible or isolated as we search for answers without outside help.

Susan Sontag observes in *Illness as Metaphor* that illnesses we don't understand are frequently viewed as manifestations of inner states. They can be written off as merely psychological and disregarded or discounted. We all deserve to be taken seriously, to be treated with dignity and believed. It is hard enough to deal with pain, and then worse to be discounted.

There is so much value placed on productivity and career success, but living with chronic pain can sometimes take up all the energy we have just to make it through the day. Finishing tasks and small accomplishments can seem like finishing a marathon. It can be uncertain on any given day whether we can rely on our bodies or energy. It is so hard to be perceived as unreliable or undependable, and we may worry that we might let others down.

Alison Lurie writes in *The Last Resort*, "Having a chronic illness, Molly thought, was like being invaded. Her grandmother back in Michigan used to tell about the day one of their cows got loose and wandered into the parlor, and the awful time they had getting her out.

That was exactly what Molly's arthritis was like: as if some big old cow had got into her house and wouldn't go away. It just sat there, taking up space in her life and making everything more difficult, mooing loudly from time to time and making cow pies, and all she could do really was edge around it and put up with it."

Discovering that we have a chronic health condition can make us feel powerless. While we can't always halt the illness in our bodies, we can seek comfort, inspiration, and support on this difficult journey. In the midst of grieving what was, perhaps we can find acceptance: a difficult life task, but so important for growth.

May the chapters in "Fall" support you in recognizing your anger and frustration and finding wisdom in present awareness. And mostly, may you know that you're not alone in this journey.

1
Letting Go

*Some people believe holding on and hanging in
there are signs of great strength. However, there
are times when it takes much more strength
to know when to let go and then do it.*

Ann Landers

Fall is a season of transformation and change, showing us the colorful glory of letting go. As the leaves flutter to the ground, they create a blanket of nourishment for new life, replenishing the soil for future growth. In our own lives, when we let go of what no longer serves us—whether it's difficult memories, worries, or outdated beliefs—we make room for new opportunities, experiences, and connections.

Being able to let go is a useful skill to cultivate for living and thriving with chronic illness. Letting go isn't only about loss; it is a process of change. There is beauty in transformation, and there can even be freedom when we release emotions like worry, fear, and anger. It can also be a powerful tool in coping with pain.

Sometimes letting go is as simple as bringing attention to your breath. As you exhale, you could focus on a thought or emotion that you wish to release. You can also focus on cultivating a different thought or emotion as you inhale. This basic breathwork can help relax the mind and body.

As we know, letting go isn't as easy as snapping our fingers. The spiritual act of letting go often involves examination and tuning into your body, thoughts, and spirit. The work can be hard, but it can ease the load when living with chronic illness and pain.

Letting Go of Ego and Certainty

Julianne's Story

I'm a youngest child, and as youngest children tend to do, I struggled with finding my identity and place within my family. One of the key identities that I claimed was strength. I was a 70s kid who grew up in the South, and my role models were Wonder Woman, Charlie's Angels, and Laura Ingalls Wilder from *Little House on the Prairie*. I wanted to be a strong, capable girl, not dependent on any boy to save the day. At the skating rink in fourth grade, I remember gleefully arm wrestling one kid after another. Who had time for skating backwards when you could win arm wrestling competitions?

Being strong and capable developed into a core part of who I wanted to be. I started restaurant work at fifteen and worked three jobs during college, and in those jobs I was always the one who was asked to open jars. It was a matter of pride that I could twist open the jar that no one else could open. In my jobs or in my personal life, capability and strength were one way to show that I could take care of myself.

In my late twenties I eventually became a massage therapist, and my hand strength became my signature for the deep, therapeutic massage that I offered. I had my own massage practice for over ten years, until I became a full-time minister. After that, I still traded massages with other practitioners.

In the heart of the pandemic, in March of 2021, I was diagnosed with rheumatoid arthritis. I had a strong onset of crippling pain in my hands along with increased swelling in my feet, and I found it difficult to do many daily tasks and struggled with the stairs in my house. As a minister, I was concerned with keeping up with my responsibilities and learning how to function through pain. During one of the scariest and most stressful periods of my life, a lot of my physical capability and strength were stripped from me. Besides the pain and discomfort, I was surprised by the emotional loss I experienced with this sudden change. I felt bereft of capability.

Even a year and a half later, I found myself miffed at the dinner table when my sixteen-year-old son was the one who could open a jar of spaghetti sauce. The next day I needed to recruit his and my spouse's help to get the garden and yard ready for winter. Late fall is unpredictable in Wisconsin; winter can come hard and fast, whether you're ready for it or not. I had intended to help put away the garden furniture, pots, and soil, but I found I had no energy left for it between full-time work and parenting. When a hard snow fell, I felt like a squirrel caught before gathering all of my winter provisions.

Luckily, two weeks after the snow, we had a Saturday with temperatures in the forties. I was able to work with my son and spouse to put away the outside furniture and prepare for the bitter cold to come. I am learning to accept help with grace and more gratitude.

Letting go of certainty, letting go of ego, letting go of the idea that I must be strong and able to control my days is a central part of my process in living with chronic illness.

Gold Leaf

by Julianne Lepp

We are the sum of our accomplishments, are we not?
Counting our worth by degrees, achievements,
and the glory of our completed tasks.

This need for achievement clings tightly,
like constricting saran wrap left on too long.
Each call, each task needs that gold star,
especially on days like these.

Days where I can only wear soft socks
and ice is my closest friend.
Nights when sleep is impossible,
doing tasks in the wee hours
and catching up on rest in the morning.

Can I keep down food
while adapting to this new medication?
Did I catch all the details in the last call?

Some days there is energy and joy
in movement. Other days,
my illness is like some invisible intruder,
stealthy and unpredictable.

On days like these,
I can't keep on pretending nothing has changed
any more than a tree can hold onto its leaves in the fall.
My bare branches are showing.

TEND TO YOUR SPIRIT

My body is telling me it is time to adapt.

What if I shed the tight bands of success
and gather the leaves of change about me?
Glorious as a tree in autumn,
with orange leaves for compassion and complexity,
yellow for caution and care,
and brilliant red for joy in the moment,
celebrating beauty as it comes.

I am not done with my changes
and change is not done with me.
I am learning to rest in uncertainty.
To accept changes I cannot control.
A gold leaf is my new gold star,
and it is enough for me.

*Are you recognizing the moments when you give
yourself grace? The moments when you're letting go
of negative self-talk and being kind to yourself?*

Give yourself a gold leaf!

The Teaching Bean

by Elizabeth Tarbox in *Evening Tide*

When I was a child my stepmother gave me and my sister each a lima bean. She showed us how to dampen some blotting paper and line a jam jar with it, and how to place the bean carefully between the blotting paper and the jar. She told us to stand the jars on the windowsill in our bedroom and keep the blotting paper wet, and watch to see what would happen.

A little later I took my bean out and polished it up with a bit of furniture polish. It was shiny now and smelled much better than my sister's bean.

In a few days my sister's bean swelled and a strong white root pushed out of the bottom of the bean. My bean just sat there. A week later my sister's bean sprouted a green shoot that forced its way up and out of the top of the jar. My bean did nothing, but began to look wrinkly. In another week my sister's jar was full of roots and shoots and the bean was ready to be planted. My bean shriveled up and fell to the bottom of the jar and I threw it away.

How often have I covered things with furniture polish to make them shiny, to make them smell better? How often in my life have I cared more about the way things look, and how they smelled, rather than how they really were? I spent half a lifetime covering my feelings with the emotional equivalent of furniture polish, thinking that if I looked good and smelled good the ache inside would go away.

But spirits are not like beans, thank God. They may shrivel with neglect, but as long as life persists there is the chance to wash off the polish and redeem the growing thing inside.

Spiritual Practice

Letting Go

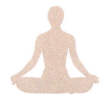

Living with chronic illness is hard, and it isn't easy to shed resentment, anger, and frustration. Sometimes we wear our pain like a badge, until it becomes an identity that we dwell within. Sometimes we cling to habits or relationships that are causing pain or harm. It is important to acknowledge our suffering, anger, and other difficult emotions. It is also important to recognize that we are not our emotions.

> We are not our feelings. We are not our moods. We are not even our thoughts.... Self-awareness enables us to stand apart and examine even the way we 'see' ourselves.
>
> STEPHEN R. COVEY

Here are three approaches to the spiritual practice of letting go. You may want to take your time over a day or a week to contemplate the relationships, habits, emotions, or ideas that are no longer serving you. If it is helpful, write down what you wish to release.

- Find some stones or other small objects, like beads or buttons, that can be held in the hand. Each one will represent something you wish to release. Fill a bowl partway with water and situate yourself where you can drop the stones into the bowl. Relax into this time that you have created for yourself and calm your breath. Take a stone, say out loud what you wish to let go, and drop it into the water. Keep doing this until you reach the end of your list. Afterward, you may also choose to burn or compost the list.

- Take a household task, like washing dishes or cleaning the bathroom. As you gather the objects you are cleaning, say aloud what you wish to let go. As you clean, imagine you are clearing away what you wish to release. Once you're done, take a moment to assess whether you feel a sense of release, and affirm it if so. This practice can be repeated until you feel the release.

- Find a song, perhaps from the Letting Go playlist, and play it in a comfortable space. Close your eyes and sink into stillness and relaxation. As the music washes over you, picture the things you wish to release. On each refrain, imagine the lightness and freedom you will feel as a result. Afterward, try to bring that sense of lightness with you into your day.

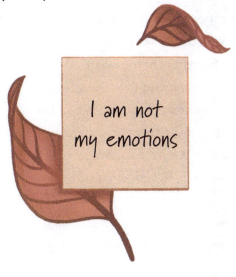

Letting Go of Expectations

Justyna's Story

I'm a single mom with three young boys, and I was diagnosed with rheumatoid arthritis several months ago. I'm also a first generation American whose parents grew up in Poland. I'm still trying to navigate what triggers my symptoms. For now, I'm trying to live life like I lived it before, just toning it down a little bit.

My mom is very understanding when I don't feel good and will take the kids for a little bit, helping them with homework or playing with them. My dad doesn't get it: my illness isn't something you can see. To him it's like, "You're not doing anything when you get home, you're just sleeping all day, or you're on the couch all day." And I'm like, "Yeah, because I hurt." I can't even open a water bottle right now. It has been a mix of both reactions in my family. I do think it is a generational thing. My parents try to understand, but it is hit or miss.

This has changed my life, though: I feel like I have to be more cautious. I'm always on the go, so it feels like a whole new world that I'm trying to figure out. At the kids' birthday at the trampoline park, I can't risk jumping and then being so sore I can't move. I used to be a cake decorator, but if I go back into that, how can I do that without hurting myself? I'm now going to school for graphic design. With my kids, if I'm having a flare, I tell them I'm sick and we're going to slow down. I've also had to slow down schooling since diagnosis.

I don't know if this illness is something I've always had, but when I had my twins, it was a rough pregnancy. After that, I noticed I became allergic to many things. I would notice my wrist and knee hurting. Then it seemed fine for about four years, but then I got Covid and it all went downhill. I ended up in the hospital for hypertension, and I couldn't even turn my head due to pain. And once the doctors had my hypertension under control, they thought I was fixed. It took months to get a referral and have my pain taken seriously. Once I was diagnosed and got medicine, I felt like I was myself again.

My advice is to basically listen to your body and listen to yourself. If you need a break, take a moment, but don't let it stop you from doing what you want to do. You might have to rework your plan and do things a little differently. For your own mental health, you don't have to put your life on hold.

From *You Don't Look Sick: My Journey with an Invisible Illness*

by Kristen Dutkiewicz

No one knows what the future holds. I know I have multiple sclerosis, and I know it is not going anywhere anytime soon. I want to make the most of every day I have because, yes, I do constantly face the fear of another relapse. Therefore, I want to cherish the days I am feeling well. However, even if someone does not have MS, or an autoimmune disease, they should also be making the most of every day!

What a gift life is!

Life can also absolutely be blindingly overwhelming, and when that happens, I need to remind myself to take one day at a time. This was my mantra as I was recovering from my relapses. It was like living a real life miracle as I witnessed myself improve just a little bit day by day, but when I just wanted everything to be "normal" again, I had to focus on how far I had come.

Little steps forward are better than no steps at all.

I have a somewhat controlling personality. I like to know what is going to happen next. I love schedules. MS also likes to be in control. Therefore, I needed to learn how to let go of a lot of control, and just let things happen.

Letting go of control is not always a bad thing.

Sometimes letting go helps you slow down. And it is OKAY to slow down.

One final piece of advice that I learned when I was only nine years old . . . something else that is okay . . .

It is okay to cry.

Crying does not make you weak. Crying makes you human! Sometimes letting loose and taking a moment to let your emotions flow is just the release you need to come back stronger than ever.

What I learned cannot be summarized or turned into a useful truism. It rather resembles a glint in the earth, a bit of mica on the rock that catches the sun just so. I'm always trying to turn to that sun, to be adrift in the snow-shine, to find the aspect that stuns me into a reverence I know I can't control. I will not say that this is the gift of illness, because I do not think illness is a gift. It is not anything so tangible and fixed. But this may be illness's reality, its weather, the way swaying underfoot is a quality of sea travel one only knows in full by stepping back, once more, on firm land.

MEGHAN O'ROURKE, *THE INVISIBLE KINGDOM*

From *Turning Suffering Inside Out: A Zen Approach for Living with Physical or Emotional Pain*

by Darlene Cohen

If you have some catastrophic change in your life, like disease or injury, one of the most difficult things facing you is letting go of the past—the easy, idyllic past—and focusing on the life you have now. It's easy to forget that even before the catastrophe, you didn't think of your life as easy. There was too much to do in too little time; you didn't see yourself as on top of things and in control, operating at peak efficiency. It is very difficult to have a strong, functional body displaced by a painful, helpless one. It shakes you to your very identity. In order to heal in this situation, you have to give up your past, to grieve your former body and then turn away, to learn to see your present body as real and your current life as demanding all the creativity and energy you can summon, maybe even more. If we have lost the relative ease and mobility of the past, it may be hard to make a real commitment to this new life. There's a tendency to deny these new circumstances and wait for our old life to return. But in every moment, every day, every week we spend lamenting our lost life, we also have an opportunity to shift all our interest and creativity to this new life. Perhaps even more than in the past, our lives demand everything we can bring to them. The purpose of our lives may not be to produce something wonderful or to become rich or famous or renowned for wisdom; the purpose may just be to express our own sincerity doing completely whatever it is we do, immersing ourselves in the situation in which we find ourselves. When our way is very hard, we have an opportunity to use every flicker of our imaginative fire. This attitude gives us a tremendous sense of freedom and creativity. We feel as if we can imbue any situation with the richness of our own poetry.

After I was bedridden with rheumatoid arthritis, my mobility was so impaired that volunteers from the San Francisco Zen Center began cleaning my room, doing my laundry, and washing my hair. As my body got weaker and my pain greater, and I could no longer deny my situation, I realized that this is the life I have been given. This is the body I have to live the rest of my life with. Within my experience, this is my reality. Every day, I woke up and began to say, "What part of my body can I use today to do the things I have to do?" Strangely, I found relief in just being the suffering. Because I was so ill, nothing was demanded of me: no function, no performance, no self-sufficiency, no heroics. Just me living and breathing. This baseline life allowed me to live in a very simple, non-demanding way.

Journal Prompts
Releasing Emotions

Chronic illness can bring a lot of difficult emotions. There can be worries over an unresolved diagnosis or medicine and frustrations over how illness will impact relationships, money, jobs, and capability. Fall can be a time to focus on releasing thoughts that are holding you back. In this journal prompt, you're invited to read the following poem by Mark Morrison-Reed and respond to the prompts below.

- What concerns and emotions are holding you back right now from living life to the fullest? What might you be ready to release and let go?

- The poet discusses taking the time to savor and appreciate life. Think about a time of laughter, beauty, or other powerful emotion and savor and remember it by writing it down.

- Take one line from the poem and expand on how it relates to your experiences with chronic illness.

Let Me Die Laughing

by Mark Morrison-Reed
from *Been in the Storm So Long*

We are all dying,
our lives always moving toward completion.

We need to learn to live with death,
and to understand that death is not the worst of all events.

We need to fear not death, but life—empty lives, loveless lives

lives that do not build
upon the gifts that each of us has been given, lives that are like
living deaths,
lives which we never take the time
to savor and appreciate,
lives in which we never pause to breathe deeply.

What we need to fear is not death,
but squandering the lives we have been miraculously given.

So let me die laughing, savoring one of life's crazy moments.
Let me die holding the hand of one I love, and recalling that I
tried to love and was loved in return. Let me die remembering
that life has been good, and that I did what I could.

But today, just remind me that I am dying so that I can live,
savor, and love with all my heart.

Reflection Questions

Letting Go

- What did your family, friends, or faith tradition teach you about letting go while you were growing up? How have your thoughts or actions around letting go remained the same or changed over time?

- Are there some emotions that you find easier to let go of than others? Why might this be?

- When you imagine releasing something, how does that make you feel in your body? When you notice physical cues in your body or experience emotional responses, what might they tell you?

- What has been a life-affirming experience of letting something or someone go?

When you experience loss, people say you'll move through the five stages of grief... Denial, Anger, Bargaining, Depression, Acceptance...
What they don't tell you is that you'll cycle through them all every day.

RANATA SUZUKI

Playlist for Letting Go

I Didn't Know My Own Strength by Whitney Houston

Dance Again by Selena Gomez

Begin by shallou

See the Sun by Dido

Can't Go Back by The Crane Wives

Part of Me by En Vogue

Let It Be by the Beatles

Make Me a Channel of Your Peace by Susan Boyle

God Is a River by Peter Mayer

2
Grief and Compassion

A true practice of grieving is like any healing. It requires
attention and patience. It takes its own time.

Carmen Ambrosio

Fall is not only a time of letting go; it is a time of grieving for what is changing. In the seasons of illness, after the first shock of a new diagnosis or a new health challenge, grief can be as much a part of our experience as any of the physical manifestations of our condition. Grief comes naturally with the huge losses that chronic pain and illness can bring, and it can accompany us for many years, darkening our days and causing immense suffering. But grief is also inseparable from the process of coming to terms with these changes. There is no way we can leap over our grief or pretend it away.

The sadness and pain that can come from the loss of health or mobility is often not recognized as grief at all. Most people think of grief as the loss of a loved one, which means that both we and those around us may not even realize that our emotions around health losses are another form of grief. Recent scientific work on grief has shown that it has measurable physiological effects throughout the body, especially in the brain, reducing our cognitive and decision-making abilities. Grief, although a natural response, has its own effects on our well-being.

In some cultures grief is downplayed, dismissed, or judged. This leads us to judge ourselves for grieving, which adds even more suffering to the suffering we are already experiencing physically. Compassion can help soften our hearts so we can feel our grief and honor it, and fully experiencing our own grief helps us to connect with compassion for others.

Finally, grief can be a spiritual practice. As Karen Hering writes in *Trusting Change*: "A true practice of grieving is like any healing. . . . It requires attention and patience. It takes its own time. It will be uniquely ours, perhaps similar to others but never identical—and sometimes wholly unlike the experience of anyone else."

In this chapter, you are invited to read stories and poetry of grief and gently explore your own relationship with grief and compassion through journal prompts, spiritual practices, and music.

> Having compassion starts and ends with having compassion for all those unwanted parts of ourselves. The healing comes from letting there be room for all of this to happen: room for grief, for relief, for misery, for joy.
>
> PEMA CHODRON

The Countries of Grief

Florence's Story

Is it possible to live each day knowing that everything will go wrong—that everything is falling apart right now—yet remembering, too, that this in no way denies the living truth, the love at the heart of existence?

SY SAFRANSKY

My marriage ended on my thirty-fourth birthday. I had spent the previous ninety days, from January to April, at Tassajara Zen Mountain Monastery, deep in the snowy Big Sur mountains, sitting in meditation for many hours each day. I had waited years to be able to do this. It was a challenging time for me, though also a powerfully joyful time.

One day while I was meeting with my Zen teacher, I told him about a story I had read when I first became interested in Buddhism and how significant it had been for me. It goes like this: Ajahn Chah was a great Thai meditation teacher. One day he was speaking to his students and he held up a glass of water. He said, "I have this beautiful water glass. The light shines through it, and it holds my water admirably. But to me this glass is already broken. I know one day it will definitely break. And I appreciate it all the more, knowing this. When I understand that the glass is already broken, every moment with it is precious."

After I shared the story, we began to talk about trust and what it means to trust another person, even when we know our time together is limited and understand all the ways we can hurt one another. He said, startling me, "Real trust includes loss and betrayal." The day I left Tassajara, after ninety days on retreat, my spouse told me that he had fallen in love with someone else and had already decided to leave our marriage. We had been together for eleven years. We loved and respected one another, and I had gone to Tassajara with his blessing. On the day I found out that my marriage was over, my life shattered. On that day I entered the country of grief.

Most people, sooner or later, travel through that strange, topsy-turvy country. Nothing I could say about it would be unfamiliar, if you've been there. I told friends that I felt like I had been hit by a truck. There was no warning, no way to brace myself. Not only did I lose my beloved and our life together, but I lost the old farmhouse we had bought together a few years before, the cat and dogs I loved, my community, the very foundations of my life. I felt like I was wandering in the woods at night, lost and keening, bumping into trees and falling down.

This went on for a long time. Six months after my marriage ended, someone told me I should be past the grief. (Please don't ever believe anyone who gives you a timeline for loss and sorrow.) At eight months, I wondered whether I would survive. Finally, more than a year later, I found a way out of that country of grief, or at least I walked toward its edge.

And then something happened to my health. Suddenly, also without warning, I was very, very sick. Most healthy 35-year-olds don't expect to become sick. It was completely bewildering. I went straight from one territory of grief—the loss of a marriage—to other territories: the loss of health and youthful vigor.

Much later I learned, in chaplaincy training, how many forms of grief there can be. We think of grief primarily as a response to the loss of a loved one, but there can be grief in any loss or transition. I remember looking at the long, long list of possible causes of grief and nodding. "Yes, yes, that's how it is." Loss of health, loss of relationship, loss of identity, loss of work or career, loss of a pet, loss of mobility, loss of capacity, loss of a home, loss of a pregnancy, loss of a possibility, loss of independence, the losses when a child grows up or a loved one ages ... When I saw that list, I recognized how many losses I had experienced in a single year of my life, and understood for the first time why the depth of the grief was so overwhelming. Unfortunately, experiencing the pain of a grief that is not culturally recognized can leave one even more isolated and bereft: few people think to send a condolence card to someone with a new medical diagnosis.

Grief can be isolating, but it can also bring us into communion with all the other people who have experienced loss. As I wrote in an essay called "Dancing in the Dark Fields: The Teachings of Illness," "I've cried a lot of tears of self-pity in the last few years, and I wonder why 'self-pity' is such a pejorative term. To feel pity for the person in pain—me—has been the first step toward really understanding that this is the human condition. Our tears mingle together, a big invisible river circling around the world, and through my tears of self-pity I join everyone who cries."

There are many reasons to cry in this life. Ajahn Chah was right about his water glass. I understand, after years of chronic illness, that this body is already broken. I try to remember now to appreciate what is still possible for me, and when tears well up in my heart for what is lost, to let them overflow, joining everyone who cries.

It's okay to grieve the losses of chronic illness. It's okay to be broken; everyone is in some way.

ALLISON ALEXANDER, *SUPER SICK*

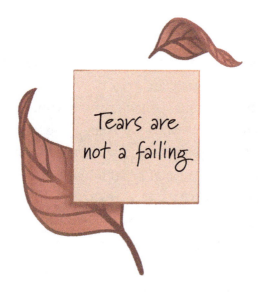

Tears are not a failing

Spiritual Practice
Self-Compassion

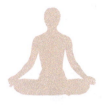

Self-compassion is simply giving the same kindness
to ourselves that we would give to others.

CHRISTOPHER GERMER

Most of us have not been taught the spiritual practice of self-compassion. Quite the opposite: we may have been told that we should never feel sorry for ourselves, even in very difficult circumstances. For this spiritual practice, you are invited to gently open to compassion for your own condition.

Find a comfortable position sitting in a chair or lying down, perhaps wrapped in a soft shawl or blanket. Take a few breaths and bring to mind the challenges of your life. These could be physical, emotional, or any other life circumstance that is causing suffering. If tears come, let them come. If anger comes, or any other emotion, allow that too. Just keep coming back to your breath and the difficulties you face. Notice if any harsh or scolding thoughts toward yourself come up, and if they do, remind yourself that your intention for this time is to offer compassion to yourself, as foreign as that may feel.

After a few minutes of breathing and connecting to what is hard in your life, offer these compassionate wishes to yourself, just as you might to someone else who is facing challenges.

May I be free from suffering
May I be at ease
May I find healing

If these phrases don't resonate with you, find others that work for you. This is an ancient Buddhist practice for cultivating compassion. If you find it difficult to feel self-compassion, just keep coming back to your difficult circumstances, caring for yourself as a dear friend or family would care for you. Continue for a few minutes.

If you want, you can expand your meditation to include others. Bring to mind or imagine other people facing similar challenges and offer them these compassionate wishes as well.

May you be free from suffering
May you be at ease
May you find healing

End by connecting to a feeling of love and care for yourself and all who are suffering.

Stray

by Florence Caplow

With thanks to "Talking to Grief" by Denise Levertov

Grief
like a large stray dog,
silent but determined
follows me through my day.
I wake up and a moment later he is at my side,
wet nose pressed against my heart.

Drinking tea, he hovers just behind me.
In the morning light of the fading garden
I think with relief that perhaps he has gone elsewhere
and then I see him lying in the shade,
his eyes fixed on mine.

I shoo him away to no avail.
He smells a little of wet dog,
of a dog who's been too long out in the rain.
I am afraid he wants to move in permanently.
A ghost, a recurring dream.

When I walk the autumn streets
he pads along,
reminding me of my sorrows
with a deep whine, a disconsolate howl
that I fear will rouse the neighborhood,
lead to petitions calling for my removal.

TEND TO YOUR SPIRIT

At night when all is still
he curls up beside me
pressing his back against mine
daring me to move away.

Oh dog of grief, everywhere you go you are unwanted.
I wish for enough kindness in my heart
to feed you, touch your rough, unwashed fur
and tell you that you are worthy
as any other being
on this sad and lovely earth.

From "A Young Widow Rewrites the Conventional Narrative of Grief"

Amy Lin, in conversation with Jared Jackson

Our language around grief is limited. One way is by this desire to make people feel better. Culturally, I think, humanly, we do not want to see our fellow people in pain. We want to make them feel better. And this is where I think, with most people, because of their good intentions, the language that they use is always forced towards healing, towards "cheer up," towards the "bright and shiny." The language we have for grief is about either distracting people from it or helping them feel better generally. And while that comes from a really human and understandable place, grief studies show it's harmful to people who are grieving because grief is chronic pain. It doesn't go away. . .

And it becomes really harmful for people who are grieving to have to perform that they're not sad. Or to perform that you've made them feel better. But it's also hard to educate gently, especially when you just want to say, "If you want to help me, please just sit with me in my sadness."

And then the second part where I see us limiting language around grief comes from, I think, a North American narrative of resilience, the bootstraps mentality, the "you're so strong." I think people see it as kind of cheerleading, truthfully. But again, it really just puts a griever in a place where there's no space for them, and nobody feels strong or resilient. They feel afraid. That's how they feel.

Each person's grief is as unique as their fingerprint. But what everyone has in common is that no matter how they grieve, they share a need for their grief to be witnessed. That doesn't mean needing someone to try to lessen it or reframe it for them. The need is for someone to be fully present to the magnitude of their loss without trying to point out the silver lining.

BRENÉ BROWN, *ATLAS OF THE HEART*

Are you able to allow yourself tears and sadness over your condition without judging yourself?

Give yourself a gold leaf!

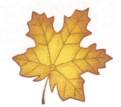

The Grief Runs Deep

Cristy's Story

I'm a white, cisgender, midlife woman, a mom, a partner, a sister, a friend, and a family nurse practitioner. And I love being in the wilderness. Wilderness touches my heart, particularly the high mountains. I have loved to be outside in all kinds of ways: on my feet, on my mountain bike, or on my skis. These things have brought me great joy and deep friendship over many years.

Because of all that, I used my body pretty hard for a long time. A few years ago something in my back started to wear out, but I kept running and being on my bike and hiking. And then suddenly it completely fell apart, on March 20th, 2021. The pain and weakness and the radical change in my ability to do things seemed to happen overnight.

Initially I thought, "Oh, surely I'll get through this." I kept working as a nurse practitioner, but the pain was excruciating. I took time off and saw three different surgeons who all said, "Fuse your lumbar spine." The surgery helped the pain, and I did everything to recover, but my ability to move or walk as I did before hasn't come back. I'm not able to do the work that was meaningful for me, and most of the things I loved to do in the wilderness are no longer possible.

In these years I have experienced a river of grief and overwhelming sadness. I have learned that sadness will come and it will go, and that's helpful. I did a meditation retreat a while ago and was reminded how important it is to just sit with the grief. It won't consume you or eat you alive, though it can feel that way.

And there's a lot to learn in that. I just try and hold things a little more lightly, if I can.

I know it's good to focus on what I can do, not what I can't, and yet the grief still runs deep. I have a meditation practice. I really try to connect with people. I try to do what I can. Journaling has been a powerful practice: a journal goes with me everywhere I go. I have needed to find other ways to ground myself and other ways to connect to mountains. One of the things I've done a lot of is go to the mountains with my partner. While he goes for a run with our dog, I walk a short distance with my book and my thermos cup, and I read in a beautiful place. We have been able to withstand this incredible challenge, and our connection has deepened and feels more solid than ever.

My advice to others around grief? Really honor your grief and everything that comes with it: despair and frustration and anger. Don't isolate. Remember, you're so much bigger than whatever disability you may have (I don't really like the word "disability"). Try to keep loving your life, enjoy the small, wonderful things that happen, and keep doing whatever brings you alive, even if it's scary.

You are who you are no matter what. For instance, I know that because of all the things I've done in the outdoor world, I'm tough and determined. I love the people in my life. I love being in nature. All these parts remain and aren't going to change. There's a bunch of things I can't do, but I will always be that person no matter what. It is really, really sad to not be able to do the things that I loved or be in the mountains the way I once could. But I'm still me.

Journal Prompts
Grief Around Illness and Pain

This is a moment of suffering. Suffering is part of life. May I be kind to myself in this moment. May I give myself the compassion I need.

KRISTIN NEFF

Think of one small thing that you have lost because of your illness or pain. There are many huge things, but for this exercise, find one small thing, maybe even a very small thing, a prosaic thing.

Perhaps this is a simple activity you did before that is no longer possible to do, or a way of feeling, or part of your identity. Maybe it's so small that you feel kind of silly naming it. Choose something around the edge of loss, not the center of it.

When you are ready, write that small loss on the top of your paper. Hold it in your mind for a while; breathe with it. If tears come, welcome them. If they don't come, just be with whatever feelings arise. Notice what you feel.

When you are ready, start writing about this loss: what it is, why it matters, what you felt as you brought it to mind and heart. Give yourself at least five minutes. Then explore the questions below in writing.

- What wisdom do you want to offer yourself around this loss?

- What would you say to a dear friend who had this loss?

- Are there any ways that this activity could still be part of your life if done in another way? What would those possible ways be?

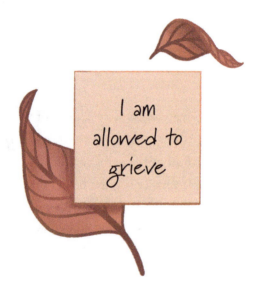

I am
allowed to
grieve

Reflection Questions
Grief

- How has grief shown up in your journey through chronic illness or pain?

- What have you learned about living with grief's unfolding, whether through other losses or around the losses that come with your own physical challenges?

- How do others respond to your grief? Do you feel supported in what you feel? Dismissed?

- How do you respond to your own grief? Are you able to honor your grief with some compassion?

> How to live when the ground has been taken away. No more mother or father, no more energy of youth, no more dream of infallibility. No more health.
>
> NATALIE GOLDBERG, *LET THE WHOLE THUNDERING WORLD COME HOME*

Playlist for Grief

In the Arms of an Angel by Sara McLachlan

Miserere mei, Deus by Gregorio Allegri, sung by Tenebrae

Ball and Chain by Willy Mae Thornton, sung by Janis Joplin

The Next Right Thing by Kristen Anderson-Lopez and Robert Lopez, sung by Kristin Bell

SING by Jon Batiste

Dante's Prayer by Loreena McKennitt

Everybody Hurts by R.E.M.

My Silver Lining by First Aid Kit

We Could Fly by Rhiannon Giddens

Calling All Angels by MaMuse

Adagio for Strings by Samuel Barber

Stabat Mater by Giovanni Battista Pergolesi

Sonata No. 8 Op. 13 "Pathétique," 2nd movement by Ludwig van Beethoven, performed by Daniel Barenboim

Spem in Alium by Thomas Tallis, sung by the Tallis Scholars

Trouble by Yusuf/Cat Stevens

On the Nature of Daylight by Max Richter

I Am Not Okay by Jelly Roll

3

Anger

A part of me will always be angry; such is the process of mourning the pieces of oneself that are lost to chronic disease.

Michael Bihovsky

Fall is a season of changes, and not all changes are easy. Shifting from the ease of summer days to the coming fall can feel jarring. The days are shortening, and the air is getting cooler. The seasonal changes signal the beginning of a school year or an end to days gardening in the sun. The changes that come with chronic illness can also feel jarring, and there can be a lot of loss, grief, and anger associated with them. Society teaches us that it is not okay to be angry, and not acknowledging anger can be damaging to our spirit.

Anger is a completely natural response to chronic illness. When you get sick, there might be people rushing in to make you feel better before you've even had a chance to feel what you need to feel. It is okay to not be okay! You might find yourself asking, "Why did this happen?" and "Why did it happen to *me*?" Trying to obtain a diagnosis, the right medication, or even an appointment with a health provider can be frustrating. When you are struggling with your health, finding answers and allies can feel like an uphill battle. You also might feel disoriented or like you are less in control of your life.

Anger is often portrayed negatively, but it can also be incredibly useful. The passion of anger can help us move through difficult moments or confront uncomfortable truths. However, anger can also be scary and hard to face. It is helpful to differentiate between our feelings and ourselves, reminding ourselves that we are not our emotions.

In this chapter you are invited to not judge your anger and to explore your feelings more deeply. Anger is a natural emotion, and it can be a useful tool. Being able to acknowledge anger is essential to being authentic with ourselves and understanding the challenges of living with chronic illness.

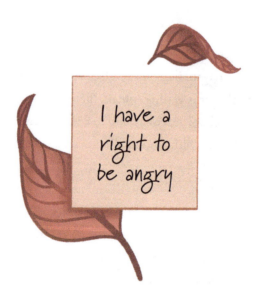

I have a right to be angry

This Is Not the Life I Planned

Julianne's Story

When I was first diagnosed with rheumatoid arthritis in 2021, I radiated with anger and disbelief. *How can this be? I'm not a sick person; this is not the future I imagined.*

For the past few years, my hands had been hurting and my feet had been swelling without explanation. I struggled with chronic insomnia and I would have sudden bouts of unexplained fevers. I was always a lot sorer than my fellow Kyuki-Do students after classes, and it took me longer to recover from sparring matches. I just thought it was middle age or a need to get in better shape. I didn't know that my body was literally fighting itself as I was sparring with my partners.

It was a great loss when I had to give up doing martial arts. The diagnosis from my family doctor caught me off guard, as he'd just congratulated me on my healthy blood pressure, good cholesterol levels, and the fact that I was in my forties and not on any prescriptions yet. At the end of this congratulatory checkup, he said, "You've been complaining for a few years about pain in your hands. Let's do a blood panel."

My happiness about my health was short-lived. The blood test showed that something was definitely wrong. He referred me to a rheumatologist, and my privileged identity as someone who was "well" was lost with my diagnosis. I didn't want to have to learn to live with pain. My image of what I could be doing in my future years was shaped by the fear of this crippling disease.

Stress is a big trigger for flares and pain in rheumatoid arthritis. The Covid pandemic was in full swing, and my symptoms skyrocketed with the pressure of full-time remote ministry and trying to keep everything together. My spiritual and emotional resources didn't seem strong enough for this huge change in my life. I began to see other caring professionals struggling with their health as well: Doctors and nurses, chaplains and teachers, and so many more reported new diagnoses and troubles. We were all barely coping with the isolation and fear.

I was angry at my body at what felt like a betrayal. I was pissed that I had a chronic illness and especially frustrated at the medicine my rheumatologist prescribed. Although it was supposed to be helping me, it made me very ill. I started with a pill form of methotrexate and found myself with painful mouth sores and nausea. When my rheumatologist switched me to injections of the same medicine, I found it difficult to give myself shots, knowing I would be left throwing up and nearly immobile with fatigue for the next twenty-four hours.

Like many with chronic illness, my pain levels and energy are unpredictable. It is frustrating to not be able to depend on my body. It is even more frustrating when people don't take my disease, pain, or fatigue seriously because they can't see it. As Eileen Davis wrote on the arthritis website CreakyJoints, "RA makes me feel angry and bitter toward people who did not support or help me when I needed it or toward those who have not shown me understanding or compassion, especially when they assume I am fine because I 'don't look sick' or I am 'too young' for my disease to be serious. I'm angry when I'm told I am fine by people who've never had to question their health like I do."

There have been moments when I have driven down empty stretches of highway and screamed out the window at the top of my lungs just to let out my frustration. I have friends who have told me that they put their anger into writing or let it out with vigorous exercise.

There are so many people dealing with the unknowns of illness, fear, and pain. The unfairness of it all makes me feel like resorting to my childhood frustration, stomping and shouting for all the people hurting: *It's not fair!* I have taken my anger out by weeding my garden until my hands and joints revolt and tell me they can do no more. Grounding my emotions in the earth gets them out of my body, each weed I toss clearing my anger and making space for calm. *Mother earth, take my anger. Mother earth, take my pain.*

Anger is a natural result of the harsh realities of chronic illness. It is powerful to give yourself the grace to experience your feelings rather than pushing them away, repressing, or ignoring them. While anger can be a motivator, a force to move you forward, it can also just be really hard. Finding outlets like writing, tears, movement, or talking with a friend or therapist can help process those feelings. I still wrestle with anger and frustration at how this illness disrupts my life and limits me. I honor my anger and try to remember that it is okay to not be okay.

From *Being Heumann: An Unrepentant Memoir of a Disability Rights Activist*

by Judith Heumann

"We're not going to let a hypocritical society give us a token education and then bury us," I told one reporter.

When it came time for my segment on *Today*, I went on completely revved up. Poor Bob Hermann. He wasn't necessarily against me, but I went after him like a dog with a bone. It was, I felt, no longer about me. It was about all the people. Yes, I did want to be a teacher, but in my mind, it was about all the stories I'd heard about someone's brother or sister, or their father, their mother, their cousin, or they themselves—and how they had this problem or that problem and no one was listening and things weren't happening. A dam had broken. After all this time, all the years of being ignored and dismissed, I felt like we had an opportunity to call attention and start to make it right. We could do something.

Spiritual Practice

Anger

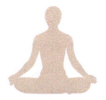

Living with chronic illness is a roller coaster, and being angry can be a natural reaction to feeling out of control. Anger can look different for each person. Some people will cry, while others will rage or seethe silently with anger. Spiritual practices can help us examine the causes of our anger and find ways to release anger in healthy ways.

It is important to recognize that anger is a natural part of being human. There is no shame in being angry.

> I have come to believe that caring for myself is not self-indulgent. Caring for myself is an act of survival.
>
> AUDRE LORDE

Here are three approaches to the spiritual practice of addressing anger:

- Take some time to examine your feelings of anger. If it is helpful, write down your thoughts. Let them flow without judgment and editing. By free writing, you may find that unexpected thoughts or emotions arise, and you may learn more about the root of your feelings. As you write, let your thoughts transfer to the page and away from your body, heart, and mind. Let the page become the receiver of your emotions and thoughts, a safe place to express yourself. Take time to care for yourself during and after this exercise.

- You may wish to physically release anger as you are able. This could be finding a safe place to shout or scream until you feel your anger is spent. It could be finding a movement that allows you to express your feelings, such as dance or moving in nature. Others express anger through painting, collage, or other art forms. Some physically release anger through burning or tearing up objects— though please do so safely.

- Find a song, perhaps one from the Anger playlist at the end of this chapter, and play it in a comfortable space. Perhaps you want to crank up the volume and let it wash over you. Or you might sing along or move as you are able to the music. You could also use music while commuting or working to release ideas or feelings that are not serving you.

Are you recognizing the moments when you are angry? Do you allow yourself time to process your emotions and find nonjudgmental support when you need it?

Give yourself a gold leaf!

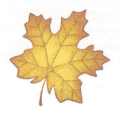

Useful Anger

by Stephen Shick in *Be the Change: Poems, Prayers & Meditations for Peacemakers and Justice Seekers*

> A good anger swallowed
> clots the blood
> to slime.
> MARGE PIERCY

But what is to be done with it,
this anger that dare not be swallowed?

Should it be diluted with denial, cooled with indifference?
Should it be sweetened with good intentions,
softened with lies?
Should it be spewed out red hot over searing tongues,
scorching the guilty and innocent alike?

What's to be done with it,
this anger that dare not be swallowed?

Don't dilute it, deny it, or cool it.
Don't sweeten it or soften it.
But, pause for a moment.

Could you hold it before your eyes
    examine it with your heart and mind?
Could you hold it
    then touch it to your belly
    that place where your soul rests?

Could you let it enter there knowing it is the part of you
    that needs to be treated kindly
    that needs to be listened to
    that needs to be honored?

For it has the power to save you,
to save us all.

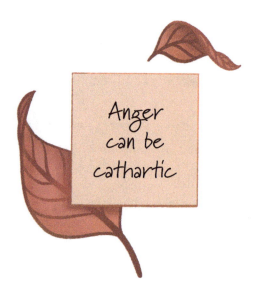

Anger
can be
cathartic

Journal Prompts

Anger

In our healing journeys, it can be important to recognize our feelings and honor each one. Although anger is often viewed as destructive or to be avoided, it can be a natural reaction when we feel out of control or overcome by hopelessness during harder times. By writing out your feelings, you may tap into ordinarily suppressed emotions and experience greater calm afterward.

To the extent that illness is a quest, it brings you to a very different place from the one you thought you were trying to get to. And so I am wary of papering over illness's real ravages with false pieties that allow us to look away from the true price exacted.

Is illness, in any way, a lesson? Illness is a travesty; illness is shit; illness is not redemptive unless it happens to be for a particular ill person, for reasons that are not replicable nor should they be said to be so. (They usually stem from the sufferer's having reached a place in the illness that makes it more bearable than it once was.) In the dark room

where I listened to life happen around me when I
was sick, I yielded a part of myself forever.

MEGHAN O'ROURKE, *THE INVISIBLE KINGDOM*

After reading the brief excerpt above, quickly write down any thoughts or feelings that arise. Has there been a time when someone tried to downplay your illness or claimed that your illness was a lesson or redemptive in some way?

You have a right to feel angry—or any other emotion that comes up for you—about your pain, loss, and illness. You have the right to draw your own conclusions about your experiences. Please be sure to practice any self-care you may need following this exercise.

Sometimes owning our pain and bearing witness to struggle means getting angry. When we deny ourselves the right to be angry, we deny our pain. There are a lot of coded shame messages in the rhetoric of "Why so hostile?" "Don't get hysterical," "I'm sensing so much anger!" and "Don't take it so personally." All of these responses are normally code for *Your emotion or opinion is making me uncomfortable* or *Suck it up and stay quiet.*

One response to this is "Get angry and stay angry!" I haven't seen this advice borne out in the research. What I've found is that, yes, we all have the right and need to feel and own our anger. It's an important human experience. *And* it's critical to recognize that maintaining any level of rage, anger, or contempt (that favorite concoction of a little anger and a little disgust) over a long period of time is not sustainable.

Anger is a catalyst. Holding on to it will make us exhausted and sick. Internalizing anger will take away our joy and spirit; externalizing anger will make us less effective in our attempts to create change and forge connection. It's an emotion that we need to transform into something life-giving: courage, love, change, compassion, justice. Or sometimes anger can mask a far more difficult emotion like grief, regret, or shame, and we need to use it to dig into what we're really feeling. Either way, anger is a powerful catalyst but a life-sucking companion.

When My Anger's Over

by Raymond John Baughan in
The Sound of Silence

When my anger's over
may the world be young again
as after rain—
the cool clean promise
and the dance
of branches glistening green.

Reflection Questions

Anger

- What did your family, friends, or faith tradition teach you about anger while you were growing up? What tools did you learn to address anger?

- How have your thoughts or actions remained the same or changed over time with how you express or deal with anger?

- From an anger management perspective, an episode of anger can be viewed as consisting of three phases: escalation, explosion, and post-explosion. Are there triggers for your anger that can be addressed before there is increased escalation? Have you used breath or mindfulness techniques to help mitigate the strength of your anger?

- Anger can give you a way to express negative feelings or motivate you to find solutions to problems. But excessive anger can cause health impacts and lead to poor decision-making. How often do you find yourself being angry? Anger can be a tool for avoidance or a response to a feeling, person, or place. What are your most typical triggers for anger?

Playlist for Anger

Seven Nation Army by The White Stripes

Believer by Imagine Dragons

Warrior by Demi Lovato

Cello Solo in C minor: The Nightmare by Basilius Alawad, performed by Martin Barman

Thunderstruck by 2Cellos

One Step Closer by Linkin Park

I Hate Going to the Doctor (The Undiagnosed Chronic Illness Song) by Kathleen Payton

Break by Three Days Grace

Boom Boom Pow by Black Eyed Peas

Redemption Song by Bob Marley and the Wailers

4

Pain

As my sufferings mounted, I soon realized there were two ways in which I could respond to my situation—either to react with bitterness or to seek to transform my suffering into a creative force. I decided to follow the latter course.

Rev. Dr. Martin Luther King Jr.

For many of us, the onset of being sick is also the onset of chronic physical pain. Like bare tree branches against a leaden sky, pain can make the body an unwelcome place. It can take many forms, from dull aches to pain so overwhelming that even moving or speaking are impossible. It can be clearly located in one part of us or diffuse. Pain is inherent in the human body, a product of our evolution. But chronic pain can drain the joy from life and leave us isolated in our suffering.

Pain can be physical or emotional, or more often than not, both. Emotional pain has a physical component, like the heavy heart of grief or the tears that fall from our eyes. Physical pain has an emotional component: like grief or anger about being in pain, or the desperate wish to find some ease.

The Buddha taught about suffering through the parable of the two arrows. The first arrow is the inevitable pain of being human and mortal: our bodies break down or we lose people we love. There is no ducking the first arrow, no matter how much spiritual practice we do. The second arrow is how we react to those difficulties. We have some choice about how we work with the second arrow, and we can find some freedom even as we still live with the realities of the first one.

For those of us with chronic pain, learning to live with its ebbs and flows is a continuous and courageous practice. Fortunately, there are resources for chronic pain: pain clinics, medications, and mind-body practices that can help us find some ease in the midst of physical pain. There is also a guided meditation on pain in the back of this book. In this chapter, you will hear first-person stories of living with pain and you will find spiritual practices, poetry, music, and journal prompts which we hope will give you inspiration and encouragement on your own journey with pain.

From *Consolations*

by David Whyte

Physical or emotional pain is an ultimate form of ground, saying, to each of us, in effect, there is no other place than this place, no other body than this body, no other limb or joint or pang or sharpness or heartbreak but this searing presence. . . .

Pain is the first proper step to real compassion. Experiencing real pain ourselves, our moral superiority comes to an end; we stop urging others to get with the program, to get their act together or to sharpen up, and start to look for the particular form of debilitation, visible or invisible, that every person struggles to overcome. In pain, we suddenly find our understanding and compassion engaged as to why others may find it hard to fully participate. . .

Lastly, pain is reluctant but unavoidable appreciation; appreciation most of all for the simple possibility of a pain-free life—all the rest is a miraculous bonus. . . Pain is a lonely road, no one can know the measure of our particular agonies, but through pain we have the possibility, just the possibility, of coming to know others as we have, with so much difficulty, come to know ourselves.

A Master Class on Pain

Florence's Story

> I think many people have a skewed idea of what "accepting" pain is. Actually, "accepting" fails to convey the tremendous energy and courage it takes to accept physical pain as part of your life. Truly accepting pain is not at all like passive resignation. Rather, it is active engagement with life in its most intimate sense.
>
> DARLENE COHEN, *TURNING SUFFERING INSIDE OUT*

About ten years after I developed an autoimmune illness, I had made plans to attend a month-long silent meditation retreat at Spirit Rock Meditation Center in California. Spirit Rock is fantastically beautiful, nestled in a valley in the hills north of San Francisco. Leaving the main road, one follows a long, winding drive lined with grassy fields and old valley oaks into the heart of the retreat center. Cars are parked in a lot outside the gates, and then the yogis, as retreatants are called, take their luggage through the gate that marks the boundary between the world of cell phones, work, family, and news and the silent world on the other side of the gates—silent except for birdsong and wind.

I had been going on Buddhist retreats for many years, but as the beginning of this one approached, I was nervous. My on-and-off-again autoimmune illness was very much "on," and I was experiencing significant pain throughout my body, like being held in a pair of vise grips. On silent retreats there is no talking, no reading, no writing, no checking email, and no cell phones. No distractions. I had big questions: If the pain continued after the retreat began, what would it be like to sit nose-to-nose with it for that long? Could I bear it?

I thought hard about whether to go, but finally decided that I would. I promised myself to take good care of my body, to practice compassion, and to be gentle with the schedule and my expectations for myself. I told myself that I could leave early if necessary.

Even though we were not supposed to bring any books with us, I decided that I would bring two fantasy novels. If the pain became overwhelming, I would allow myself to read one or both of them, as a sort of "break glass in case of emergency" approach to the rules about no reading on retreat.

I knew that every retreat has a different flavor, and there was no way to know what it would be like before I experienced it. After I arrived, despite fervently longing that my pain would recede, I continued to be in significant pain for the whole month. At the end of that time, I felt that I had been in a master class on pain.

It was not all pain; there was joy too. I was grateful for the depth of retreat practice. I thoroughly appreciated the beauty there, as the first spring wildflowers bloomed in the hills. But mostly, I practiced with pain. In a long retreat it is possible for one's awareness to become almost microscopic, and so I microscopically studied the nature of pain in my own body and experience.

I had been living with pain for ten years before the retreat, and I thought I understood it and accepted it. But as I paid attention to my experience, I realized that what I had called acceptance was closer to endurance—I was enduring pain, with my teeth gritted. And I had never noticed the difference.

There is a teaching in early Buddhism that there are three—and only three—possible responses to a sense experience, whether it is the experience of biting into a dark chocolate brownie or the pain of a sprained ankle: pleasant, unpleasant, and neutral. These responses are hard-wired into us as a part of our biology. What happens after that initial response, though, is more of a choice.

Typically, we don't consciously choose our secondary response. The usual pattern, microseconds after the initial response, goes something like, "Yum, I want more!" or "Yuck, make this experience go away," or simply "This is okay."

What I discovered on the retreat was that when I thought of my physical pain as *pain*, it was like a huge monster threatening my life. But when I thought *unpleasant* rather than *pain*, I was much less reactive to it. It was simply an experience. The next moment might well be very pleasant (though, sadly, they didn't serve chocolate brownies on the retreat).

When the sensation was *unpleasant* there was a possibility of true acceptance rather than teeth-gritted endurance, and this experience was much softer and more compassionate. It was a revelation.

These insights, and others gained on this retreat, allowed me to describe the experience of my illness at a much more granular level to my medical/healing team, and led to a genuine breakthrough in my treatment that put me in remission for years. So that master class in pain was well worth it.

(And in case you are wondering, I did read one of the books, very mindfully, during a particularly overwhelming period. Hooray for a good fantasy novel!)

Spiritual Practice

Becoming a Connoisseur of Pleasure

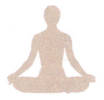

> As a person with a chronic illness who works with other people who have long-term physical difficulties, I'm very interested in what we do that has some influence on our healing process. Over the years, I've noticed that among the most important healing experiences we can have are experiences of deep pleasure.
>
> DARLENE COHEN

Darlene Cohen was a Zen student and a mother of a young child when she was diagnosed with rheumatoid arthritis in her early thirties. She later became a teacher for others in chronic pain, and she developed a unique teaching approach she called Suffering and Delight.

Her theory was that if pain is a strong component of our life experience, we also need to become connoisseurs of pleasure. She would describe entering a room and consciously noticing the sources of pleasure there—the soft blanket over a chair, the face of a beloved friend, a beautiful painting on the wall—and expanding her awareness to include these pleasures as well as whatever pain she felt. As she would say, "If you are aware of three things, and one of them is excruciating pain, the pain is going to be very large. If you are aware of a hundred things, and one of them is pain, it will be just one thing in a big field of pleasure and awareness."

Practice noticing what gives you pleasure in the ordinary things around you. Use all your senses—sight, hearing, touch, smell, taste. What is beautiful? What is soft? What smells wonderful? What happens when you open up your senses this way? If you have pain, do you notice anything about how this practice affects the experience of pain? Try this as often as you can for a week—or longer. This is a deceptively simple and powerful spiritual practice.

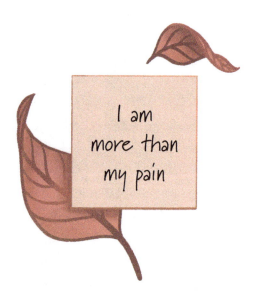

I am
more than
my pain

From "French Chocolates"

by Ellen Bass in *Like a Beggar*

But for the ill, for you with nerves that fire
like a rusted-out burner on an old barbecue,
with bones brittle as spun sugar,
with a migraine hammering like a blacksmith

in the flaming forge of your skull,
may you be spared from friends who say,
God doesn't give you more than you can handle
and ask what gifts being sick has brought you.

May they just keep their mouths shut
and give you French chocolates and daffodils
and maybe a small, original Matisse,
say, *Open Window, Collioure*, so you can look out
at the boats floating on the dappled pink water.

Life Is About Love, No Matter What

Carl's Story

I'm a cisgender male of European origin in my late seventies. I've been married for fifty-one years—I wouldn't be alive without the love of my wife, Barbara. I worked as an engineer on the Washington State Ferries before retirement. In my late forties I learned that I have spondyloarthritis, a form of reactive arthritis that usually shows up in the spine. It's different for different people. My back, my shoulders, and my wrists are all affected. I'm multi-titanium now. I've had thirteen surgeries: my whole spine is fused.

When I was home recovering from my last spinal surgery, one of my vertebrae cracked in half and cut off my spinal cord. I lost all feeling in my legs. It was during Covid, so I was all alone in the hospital. And then I developed sepsis, and then a fungal infection, and nearly died. I had to decide whether it was worth it to still live. I did, because of the people I love.

I've accepted what's going on with me a long time ago. It's important to be realistic. I know that what I have is genetic and it's not going to go away, and I have to do the best I can with what I have. As it progressed, I continued to be as active as I could. Some of that caused me damage, but on the other hand, it kept me alive mentally.

Recentering myself is very important. For me that might not look like meditation, but just being out by the beach when nobody's around and I hear the birds. And when we're talking about pain, if you don't know that part of you—that centered part, the inner part—the pain will kill you mentally. It's like you're always on the front line running for your life. So this is important, to develop ways of connecting with your deeper self.

With pain, they always ask you "One to ten, what are you feeling?" To me, a ten is when the pain is so severe that I pass out. I've been there. At pain levels two to six, I can carry on a conversation, and in fact two to four is where I am most of the time. At five or six I'm having trouble focusing on people around me and what's going on. When I get to seven or eight, I'm having trouble talking to you. I don't hear everything you're saying to me. And nine means I can't communicate. If the pain is so severe that I can't communicate with those I love, that's when pain medications become important, though I don't like how they make me feel.

Here's my advice: number one, accept that you have the pain. Number two, you're going to have to learn that you may need stronger medication for it. Don't take addictive meds like opioids to feel happy or have no pain. Take them just enough to reduce the pain where you can talk, where you've forgotten the pain for a minute or two minutes, then that's enough, and right away start tapering down the meds. Addiction is real.

Remember, this is a part of your life. There's no magic bullet. You need to accept that this is who I am and what it is now, and ask yourself, "How am I going to function and smile and have a good time despite the pain?" And that will happen. You can do that, right?

And don't hide out and turn away from people. Because life is about love. I know that from being close to death. I'm not afraid of dying now. To me, I'm a part of everything. And the blessing for me is that I get to be aware of that. That is a miracle to me; that is fantastic.

Chronic pain patients hide it so well, you can't go on how they look on the outside. They have to learn to function with pain, you can't just roll around on the floor all day screaming in agony. Medical personnel in hospitals don't even realize this. A chronic pain patient can function with a level of pain that would incapacitate any other person.

ANONYMOUS

Did you remember to take a moment to look for pleasure or beauty today?

Give yourself a gold leaf!

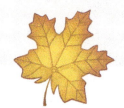

Journal Prompts

I used to think healing meant ridding the body and the heart of anything that hurt. It meant putting your pain behind you, leaving it in the past. But I'm learning that's not how it works. Healing is figuring out how to coexist with the pain that will always live inside of you, without pretending it isn't there or allowing it to hijack your day. Love the life you have.

DARLENE COHEN

Choose one or more of these prompts to explore in writing.

- Everyone with chronic pain has a pain story: how it began, what has helped or made it worse, and how it has changed over months or years. What is yours? Consider writing this story as if to a dear and unjudgmental friend.

- What practices or approaches have most helped you to live with the pain and suffering you experience? Meditation, yoga, self-hypnosis, creativity, distraction, medication? Make a list that you can refer to when you are feeling overwhelmed.

- Consider how the pain you have experienced, physical or emotional, has helped you to understand and feel compassion for others. Do you respond differently now when you see someone walking slowly toward the doors of the grocery store? Or when a friend receives a difficult diagnosis? Spend a few minutes reflecting and writing on this.

It's like a mother, when the baby is crying, she picks up the baby and she holds the baby tenderly in her arms. Your pain, your anxiety is your baby. You have to take care of it. You have to go back to yourself, to recognize the suffering in you, embrace the suffering, and you get a relief.

THICH NHAT HANH

Reflection Questions

- How has pain shown up in your life? Physical pain? Emotional pain?

- What wisdom has come your way as you have lived with pain?

- What would you advise someone who is new to chronic pain?

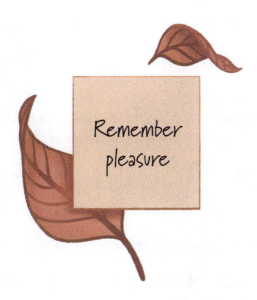

Remember pleasure

Playlist for Times of Pain

Be Like Water by Lo Wolf

Hymn of Healing by Beautiful Chorus

All Will Be Well by Meg Barnhouse

Great Compassion Chant by Plum Village monastics

Heart Sutra at Ikkyu-Ji Temple, chanted by Kanho Yakushiji

Nisi Dominus by Antonio Vivaldi, performed by Tim Mead and Les Accents

Prologues I, performed by Rodrigo Rodriguez

Agnus Dei by Samuel Barber, sung by VOCES8

William Ackerman Collection 1 by William Ackerman

Berceuse in D-Flat Major, Op. 57 by Frédéric Chopin, performed by Bertrand Chamayou

Come Healing by Leonard Cohen

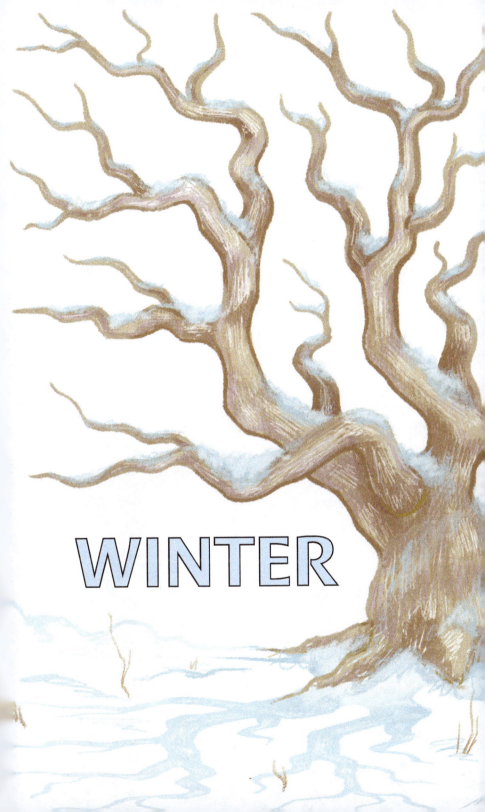

WINTER

WINTER

By Florence Caplow

The great Kentucky poet and farmer Wendell Berry wrote, in "To Know the Dark":

> To go in the dark with a light is to know the light.
> To know the dark, go dark. Go without sight,
> and find that the dark, too, blooms and sings,
> and is travelled by dark feet and dark wings.

I memorized this short poem many years ago, and each winter solstice it comes back to me, along with memories of solstice bonfires, of jumping into the icy waters of Puget Sound on that darkest night of the year, and of gatherings where the poetry of dark and of winter was passed around the circle like water-smoothed stones, hand to hand.

We experience winter in the outer world, although how it feels and looks may vary depending on where we live. And then there is winter of the body and heart, which can happen in any outer season. There comes a time, after the first shock and disbelief of a new medical diagnosis or physical challenge, after the first limitations—a pain that does not ease in the way we expected, a fatigue that does not lift—when the reality of not just *getting sick* but *being sick* begins to creep in, like days that grow gradually colder and shorter.

In my case, it took almost two years after getting sick in my mid-thirties to let in the reality of being sick, because my autoimmune illness, which came on after a bad bout of mononucleosis, was episodic, with a pattern of relapse and remission. Every time I felt fine again, even for a few days, I would think, "Great, I'm well. That was just a bad patch." And then the searing pain and weakness and nausea would return, and I would wonder why I had fooled myself again into thinking it was gone.

After two years I could no longer duck the truth, and I began, for the first time, to acknowledge that I was living with a chronic illness, one that was having profound and disabling effects on every aspect of my life. I experienced much the same pattern before I was diagnosed with rheumatoid arthritis, more than twenty years later.

Coming to terms with chronic illness can feel like sinking down through cold waters so murky you can't see your hand in front of your face. This is the time of sadness and despair, where the future can look bleak beyond imagining, like a frozen tundra as far as the horizon. This can be a time of profound isolation. The isolation is made more intense by the subjectivity of pain and illness—no one can quite know our experience, even those who love us the most. So we trudge onward, alone, maybe lost, despairing of the future, grieving our lost life. Winter in the heart.

And yet, there are ways of living and practicing with the hard-edged sword of winter. After the leaves have fallen, the bones of the world are visible, like tree branches against the winter sky. There is no hiding in winter. I have found that there is certain power and strength in saying to myself, "This is true. I may not like the circumstances of my life, but this is what it is." It's like sinking down through murky water and then finding your feet on solid bedrock. Part of what happened in my own life, when I began to truly accept that I was chronically ill, was that I got much more serious about addressing it and changing my life in response to it. My feet were planted in the reality of my situation.

The British author Katherine May, in *Wintering: The Power of Rest and Retreat in Difficult Times*, writes:

> Perhaps through all those years at school, or perhaps through other terrors, we are taught to ignore sadness, to stuff it down into our satchels and pretend it isn't there. As adults, we often have to learn to hear the clarity of its call. That is wintering. It is the active acceptance of sadness. It is the practice of allowing ourselves to feel it as a need. It is the courage to stare down the worst parts of our experience and commit to healing them the best we can. Wintering is a moment of intuition, our true needs felt keenly as a knife.

In northern Europe and Scandinavia, winters are particularly long and ferocious and daylight is very limited. The Scandinavian practice of *hygge* developed in response to these challenging winters. Hygge is the spiritual practice of finding companionship and coziness in the midst of winter, in the simplest of things around us: a cup of coffee, a warm blanket, candles and firelight. This concept can be applied to the winter of chronic illness or pain as well. Can we find comfort and ease even while in pain? Can we find comfort close by, in the day-to-day moments of our lives?

In this section, you will find reflections, meditations, spiritual practices, stories, and quotes on winter's challenges and ways of practicing with them: connecting with your innate strength, truth, and grit and finding ways to soothe and ease your heart through invoking pleasure, connection, and comfort.

5

Fear

Having courage does not mean that we are unafraid.
Having courage and showing courage means we face our
fears. We are able to say, "I have fallen, but I will get up."

Maya Angelou

In Wisconsin, winter can barge even into fall months like late October or November. It is not unusual to see children with coats over their Halloween costumes, trick or treating in the freezing temperatures. When the temperatures range up and down, the roads and sidewalks are dangerously icy, and the glory of fall can quickly turn into a slushy, brown mess. Or there might be a big snowstorm that blows in with inches upon inches of snow. Winter sweeps its wand across the world, covering everything with glistening white. All is beautiful and new.

Winter is an immersive experience in these northern latitudes. There is a breathtaking beauty to winter, the way new snow crunches beneath your boots or frost creates patterns of ice on your window. The drifts of snow cover evergreens like something out of a Christmas card.

Winter is beautiful, but it can also be incredibly difficult. For many, winter means colder temperatures, shorter days, and busy holidays. Anxieties and fears can feel more palpable with less sunlight and activity. There can also be less support and community during this season, and it can be challenging to get around in the cold and icy weather. This season can increase fears of falling, limited mobility, and susceptibility to illness.

Fear and anxiety challenge everyone, but especially those living with the complications of disability, chronic illness, and pain.

Fear—and the anxiety it creates—is one of the first emotions we encounter when we're confronted with a chronic illness. There are worries of losing independence, financial or job security, and identity and relationships. There are fears of the unknown and not knowing where to find help. Living with uncertainty is frightening. Will treatments work? Will there be a correct diagnosis? What does the future hold?

Even when fear and anxiety are overwhelming, there can still be comfort and relief. Connection with loved ones, supportive community, professional support, or our own inner resources can be a life preserver in difficult times. In this chapter we explore the fears and anxieties that arise when living with chronic illness and offer tools and hope to give support along the way.

> Life meanders like a path through the woods. We have seasons when we flourish and seasons when the leaves fall from us, revealing our bare bones. Given time, they grow again.
>
> KATHERINE MAY, *WINTERING*

This Is How We Are Called

by Kimberly Beyer-Nelson in
How We Are Called: A Meditation Anthology

In the hours before the birds
stream airborne
with chiming voice,
a silent breath rests in the pines,
and upholds the surface of the lake
as if it were a fragile bubble
in the very hand of God.

And I think,
this is how we are called.

To cup our hands and hold
this peace,
even when the sirens begin,
even when sorrow cries out, old and gnarled,
even when words grow fangs and rend.

Cupped hands
gently open,
supporting peace
like the golden hollow of a singing bowl,
like the towering rim of mountains
cradling
this slumbering and mist-draped valley.

Deprogramming Fear

Julianne's Story

Fear is an insidious emotion. Sometimes you don't notice it until it sneaks up on you at the worst possible time. One of the fears that I have had since my diagnosis of rheumatoid arthritis is navigating ice during Wisconsin winters. For healthy and able-bodied people, Wisconsin winters can be a challenge. When I'm struggling with swelling feet, concentration issues due to insomnia, or pain due to the cold, I must especially focus on my footing as I walk through icy and snow-filled parking lots and sidewalks.

Two years ago, I took a fall in a hospital parking lot, of all places, and it tumbled me into an often-unreasonable anxiety every time I had to walk outside. It made me want to bubble wrap myself to avoid any injury to an increasingly challenged body. While bracing against the cold, I had to also prepare my emotions for the possibility that I might injure myself. It took a while to work through the power that fear held on me.

Fear can also be a useful emotion. As a child, I had a great time whitewater rafting the Nantahala River in North Carolina. A couple of summers ago during a family vacation, I was offered an opportunity to raft on the river again. My first response was one of fear. I was afraid of falling out of the raft and hitting the rocks. How would my arms feel after eight hours in a boat, paddling and trying to hold on and avoid falling into the water?

It was tempting to go anyway; I didn't want to miss the beautiful mountain views and the experience of this adventure in nature. But I passed on the whitewater rafting and instead spent time with my son and dad enjoying a gentle walk and making Brunswick stew together. I felt good about listening to the wisdom of my body and moving into an acceptance of another type of joy that I could experience instead.

Living with chronic illness can be dominated by fear. How long will I be well? Can I count on my body to support me when I need to work a long day or drive on a road trip? Will my medicines work? There is so much uncertainty with illness, and learning to live with fear is one of my biggest ongoing challenges. I know many others that struggle with managing fear while trying to stay well.

The wisest teacher that I have found is my own body. When I ask myself whether my fear is justified, my body often knows the answer. If I'm overworking or overdoing it, fear and anxiety will come more easily. If I am rested and honoring the balance I need in life as well as I can, I can keep my fears and anxieties in perspective. Fear will not dominate my life.

In *The Nap Ministry's Rest Deck*, a set of practices designed to help readers disengage from grind culture, Tricia Hersey writes,

> You don't need permission from anyone to rest and listen to your body. Let your body be your teacher. Your body knows the way. Your body holds messages of liberation that I can only offer to you while you are in a rested state. One of the deepest lessons as you deprogram from the false teaching of grind culture will be learning to activate your inherent power as a human being. Your brainwashing regarding rest is intimately tied to your self-worth. You deserve rest.

Not only do we all deserve physical rest, but we deserve mental rest from pervasive fear and anxiety. We deserve a life where fear and anxiety don't rule the day.

Spiritual Practice

For Fear

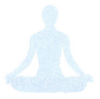

In this practice, you are invited to find a quiet and restful space. Perhaps you can use a yoga mat or lay quietly on your bed. This will be a practice of tuning into your body and allowing yourself to acknowledge any emotions that may arise. Read one or both of these quotes to yourself and then close your eyes.

> One young woman I interviewed noted, 'The emotional journey has been as hard as the physical one. The fear I feel, in combination with busy doctors who don't have time to listen, has really affected me.'
>
> MEGHAN O'ROURKE, *THE INVISIBLE KINGDOM*

> Most people live in fear of some terrible event changing their lives, the death of a loved one or a serious illness. For the chronically ill, this terrible event has already happened, and we have been let in on an amazing secret: You survive. You adapt, and your life changes, but in the end you go on, with whatever compromises you have been forced to

make, whatever losses you have been forced to endure. You learn to balance your fears with the simple truth that you must go on living.

JAMIE WEISMAN, *As I Live and Breathe*

Notice any emotions that may arise and how they feel in your body. Fear can be felt emotionally, physically, and spiritually. What are some of the fears that you might be experiencing right now about your illness or pain? What questions could you ask about that fear?

One question to ask about a fear is whether it is true. Exploring your fears and asking questions can give you a way to put things into proportion and gain a sense of agency. Tend to any needs that may arise with support from a friend, spiritual advisor, or professional counselor.

Are you noticing the moments when you are free from fear and anxiety? Are you practicing self-care in the moments when you are experiencing fear?

Give yourself a gold leaf!

From *What Doesn't Kill You: A Life with Chronic Illness—Lessons from a Body in Revolt*

by Tessa Miller

I'd battled anxiety for most my life—and continue to—but after my diagnosis and first hospitalization it made itself undeniable through panic attacks. Turns out, I learned through therapy and chronic illness support groups, that a lot of other people experience anxiety as they grieve. Claire Bidwell Smith wrote an entire book about it called *Anxiety: The Missing Stage of Grief.* "There's a multitude of emotions that come with grief. They can come up quickly and that can be scary," she said. "People often tamp those feelings down and that's one of many reasons anxiety pops up."

The solution? Allow yourself to *feel.* Sounds easy, doesn't it? Well, if you're like me, it isn't. Vulnerability wasn't rewarded as I grew up and feelings were not spoken aloud. . . . Turbulent feelings scared me, and I came to think of *all* emotions as unsafe. I put off going to therapy for so long partly because I was afraid to cry during a session. (I did cry. My psychiatrist handed me a box of tissues. The world kept turning.) Allowing myself the space and time to *feel,* even for an hour-long therapy session, seemed indulgent at first. But these thoughts subsided as I began to unpack why I felt that way, and as I started to see and feel real progress from therapy and medication.

From *Beyond the Mailbox: A Life With Chronic Illness*

by Pat Gavula

When someone is diagnosed with an illness, especially if it becomes chronic, and especially if the person diagnosed is young, many people react with a combination of sympathy and fear. Sympathy is easy to understand. Fear takes some exploring. Some fear stems from concerns for the welfare of the ill person. Will the person be able to continue working, earn a living, live a long life, engage in hobbies, ever be well again? Another fear is completely turned in on the self. This is the fear that drives friends, family, neighbors, coworkers away. This is the fear that if they get too close to a person who is ill, they might get sick too.

There is also the fear of facing one's own mortality. We all know we will die someday but for many that day is some nebulous date in the, hopefully, distant future. Hearing of the illness of a close friend or relative brings us front and center with the fact that this, too, could happen to me, and, in fact, will likely happen to me.

Fault Line

by Robert R. Walsh in *Noisy Stones*

Did you ever think there might be a fault line
passing underneath your living room:
a place in which your life is lived in meeting
and in separating, wondering
and telling, unaware that just beneath
you is the unseen seam of great plates
that strain through time? And that your life, already
spilling over the brim, could be invaded,
sent off in a new direction, turned
aside by forces you were warned about
but not prepared for? Shelves could be spilled out,
the level floor set at an angle in
some seconds' shaking. You would have to take
your losses, do whatever must be done
next.

When the great plates slip
and the earth shivers and the flaw is seen
to lie in what you trusted most, look not
to more solidity, to weighty slabs
of concrete poured or strength of cantilevered
beam to save the fractured order. Trust
more the tensile strands of love that bend
and stretch to hold you in the web of life

that's often torn but always healing. There's
your strength. The shifting plates, the restive earth,
your room, your precious life, they all proceed
from love, the ground on which we walk together.

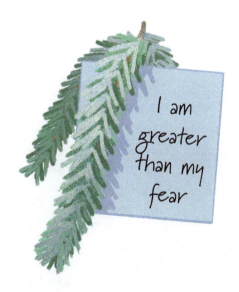

Journal Prompts

Fear

Fear can be overwhelming. These journal prompts encourage you to gently probe your fears, asking questions and letting your responses uncover hidden or unexpected aspects in a slow and safe manner.

Find a comfortable and comforting place to explore these questions. Maybe you'd like to take your time and explore this topic for a week or more. Each day, you could prepare a cozy and safe space to think about and respond to these questions. Take care of yourself and take the time you need. There is no rush or expectation with these journal prompts.

- What is my fear? Where does my fear come from?

- What does fear feel like in my body? In my heart? In my mind?

- Am I afraid of loss of control? What does losing control look like? Where do I have control and independence? What helps me feel in control?

- How do I handle my fears? What are ways in which I can put my fears and anxieties in perspective?

- What supports me when I am afraid, what tools are available to me when I have fears?

- What are some of my smallest fears? What are some of my biggest fears? Are some of these fears bigger than they ought to be as I examine them? What gives me perspective and comfort when I am afraid?

- How does my fear help me? What are the ways in which fear can be a positive?

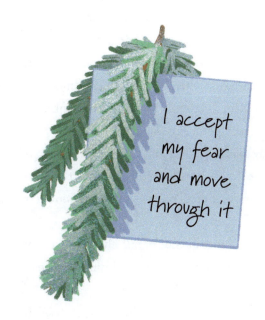

From *Fear: Essential Wisdom for Getting Through the Storm*

by Thich Nhat Hanh

Most of us experience a life full of wonderful moments and difficult moments. But for many of us, even when we are most joyful, there is fear behind our joy. We fear that this moment will end, that we won't get what we need, that we will lose what we love, or that we will not be safe. Often, our biggest fear is the knowledge that one day our bodies will cease functioning. So even when we are surrounded by all the conditions for happiness, our joy is not complete.

We think that, to be happier, we should push away or ignore our fear. We don't feel at ease when we think of the things that scare us, so we deny our fear away. "Oh, no, I don't want to think about that." We try to ignore our fear, but it is still there.

The only way to ease our fear and be truly happy is to acknowledge our fear and look deeply at its source. Instead of trying to escape from our fear, we can invite it up to our awareness and look at it clearly and deeply.

We are afraid of things outside of ourselves that we cannot control. We worry about becoming ill, aging, and losing the things we treasure most. We try to hold tight to the things we care about—our positions, our property, our loved ones. But holding tightly doesn't ease our fear. Eventually, one day, we will have to let go of all of them. We cannot take them with us.

Reflection Questions

Fear

I am afraid. Not of life, or death, or nothingness, but of wasting it as if I had never been.

DANIEL KEYES, *FLOWERS FOR ALGERNON*

- What am I afraid of? How can I challenge unhelpful thoughts?

- Is there a time when fear has been helpful to you?

- What do I need to feel safe? What can help me move through my fears?

- What support and resources help you with fear and anxiety?

Playlist for Fear

Demons by Imagine Dragons

Ocean Eyes by Billie Eilish

Bridge Over Troubled Water by Simon & Garfunkel

Till We Get the Healing Done by Van Morrison

Three Little Birds by Bob Marley and the Wailers

A Change Is Gonna Come by Sam Cooke

Come Healing by Leonard Cohen

There Is a Love, words by Rebecca Parker, music by
Elizabeth Norton

You'll Never Walk Alone by Rodgers and Hammerstein,
sung by Brittany Howard

Closer to Fine by Indigo Girls

All Will Be Well by Meg Barnhouse

Light of a Clear Blue Morning by The Wailin' Jennys

Let Me Be Brave by Beautiful Chorus

You See My Wings by Lacey Heward

6

Isolation and Connection

Take courage friends.

The way is often hard, the path is never clear,

and the stakes are very high.

Take courage.

For deep down, there is another truth:

you are not alone.

Wayne Arnason

In the depths of winter, if we live in northern climates, people tend toward hibernation and turning inward as the storms rage outside. Chronic pain and illness can similarly limit our engagement with the world beyond the walls of our home. Perhaps we are prone to infection, and in the era of Covid we fear gathering with others. Perhaps we experience severe fatigue, and so we simply don't have the physical energy to leave the house. Perhaps our physical challenges limit our mobility, and so even simple forays take a kind of effort that those who can move easily can barely imagine.

Isolation and loneliness are huge forces in the lives of almost everyone with chronic illness, especially for those of us who live alone. Even if we have loving friends and family, our condition may be hard for others to understand.

There is also the isolation of feeling alone in our suffering. However, the truth is that whatever illness we have, no matter how rare, there are other human beings who are also experiencing that illness. Whatever troubles we have, no matter how excruciating or complicated, there are other human beings who have also experienced that trouble. This is why illness-specific support groups and online forums can be so powerful. They are a reminder that our suffering is human suffering and that we are in this together. There are also Tibetan Buddhist practices where the practitioner dedicates their suffering to the well-being of others with the same condition, as another way to open the heart to our shared humanity.

Needing help, and asking for help, are great challenges for many of us, especially in a culture that celebrates independence. Learning how to ask for help is not easy, and yet it can lead to feeling less alone.

Even in a life that feels very limited, there is the possibility of finding connection, whether to other people, with the natural world, with God or Spirit, or with our own inner life. In this chapter, we explore both the painfulness of isolation and ways that connection can still be possible.

One of the hardest parts of living with chronic pain is the loneliness that comes from the repeated sense that other people don't understand what we're going through. Acknowledging to ourselves—with caring and by witnessing—how hard this is and how alone we feel starts to calm the anxious and contracted nervous system. We begin to give ourselves what we wish from others: kindness, compassion, and presence.

CHRISTIANE WOLF, *OUTSMART YOUR PAIN*

Deep Freeze

Florence's Story

It's 2 degrees Fahrenheit today in Central Illinois, and last night it was -10. The streets and sidewalks are covered in ice. I don't dare take my biodiesel car out of the garage for fear the biodiesel will gel. And I am in the fifth week of recovering from Covid, which I have already had once before. As a person on immune-modulating drugs, Covid is a rough road for me.

I spent nearly twenty days in isolation this time due to a rebound, and between the weather and my continued symptoms, I am still functionally in isolation. My doctor explained to me that the Covid vaccines are probably not as effective for me as they are for others. Ah, the life of a person with an altered immune system!

Loneliness and isolation are not usually considered symptoms of chronic illness. But nearly everyone I know with illness or chronic pain experiences isolation to some degree, and for some it is agonizingly painful. Even if one is surrounded by loved ones, loneliness can still be present, because no one else can quite know what our experience is like.

The Covid pandemic brough the whole world into isolation, with catastrophic effects on mental health everywhere. But for those of us with chronic illness, it only exacerbated the isolation we were already living. For instance, for most people now, years after the start of the pandemic, Covid is not much more than an unpleasant cold, and so the elaborate precautions of previous years are almost entirely out the window. But for me, and for many people I know, it is a different story.

I'm lucky that I can more or less support myself with online freelance work these days. Earlier in my journey with chronic illness, when I was working in an office environment full time, I experienced intense isolation because I had so little energy left after an eight-hour day. While others might have been going to hear music and spend time with friends, I was recovering from my work. My work is physically easier now, but because it is online it creates another kind of isolation. I spend much of each day in intimate connection with others, but only through a screen.

I don't know what the answer to this is. I still have limited energy at the end of many workdays, and I also need to wear a mask in crowds, which is seen as increasingly odd. Being the only person with a mask is its own kind of isolation. Yet I am experiencing the consequences of not wearing a mask right now.

One friend with chronic illness suggested that perhaps in the winter we need to think of ourselves like the animals who hunker down against the cold, out there in the woods and fields beneath the snow. In the milder months we can cavort with others, but in the winter we stay close to home, like the squirrels in their nests in the trees, quiet and snug, with our tails wrapped around our noses. Perhaps I need to embrace seasonality and the rhythms of the natural world, rather than longing for a life that is not in alignment with this body and its frailties.

Contact

by Gordon B. McKeeman
in *To Meet the Asking Years*

I stretch forth my hand
　Knowing not what I shall touch...
　　A tender spot,
　　An open wound,
　　Warmth,
　　Pulsing life,
　　Fragile blossoms,
　　A rock,
　　Ice.

I am tentative, trembling...
　Wishing to avoid hurt,
　Wanting to link my life with Life.
　　Lonely, I desire companions
　　Naked, I long for defenders.
　Lost, I want to find...
　　to be found.
　Will I touch strangers
　　Or enemies
　　Or nothing?

My hand is withdrawn
　But still it touches
　　My vulnerable skin, my furrowed brow,
　　My empty pocket, my full heart.

Do others reach, tremble, withdraw?

Do they desire, long, seek?

Are they lonely, fearful, lost?

Will they grasp a tentative, trembling hand?

I stretch forth my hand

   Knowing not what I shall touch...

   But hoping...

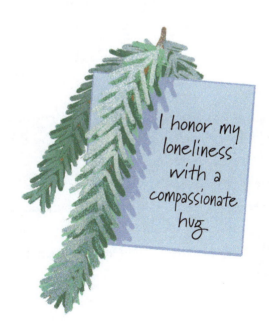

I honor my loneliness with a compassionate hug

From *Outsmart Your Pain: Mindfulness and Self-Compassion to Help You Leave Chronic Pain Behind*

by Christiane Wolf

We are social creatures that need to feel understood, seen, and heard. Because of this, our relationships with other people are critical to how we work mindfully with ongoing pain. . . .

When the internal noise level of the pain becomes incredibly loud, it drowns out everything else and we stop listening to others. We may start to hear and see those close to us through the lens of our own pain, which makes their actions seem careless or disrespectful of our feelings. Disconnection and loneliness deepen.

There are other factors that cause people who suffer from chronic pain to be more prone to isolation: feeling like nobody understands what you're going through; needing to spend more time with doctors and other health care providers; requiring lots of time for physical therapy simply to be able to get through the day; being tired because of the pain and the work it takes to "manage" it, which results in not having the time or energy to meet with friends or go out much at all. . . .

It's not your fault that your pain led to isolation, so please don't blame yourself! Offer yourself the kindness and understanding you would like from others.

Spiritual Practice
Meditation on Care and Connection

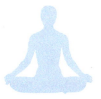

Adapted from Buddhist loving-kindness practice

For this meditation, start by sitting or lying down in a comfortable position, perhaps wrapped in a shawl or blanket, and close your eyes.

Take a few deeper breaths, if that is comfortable for you, imagining the breath moving in and out of the heart area. You could even put your hand on your heart. Feel the earth supporting you, beneath your feet or under your back.

Now think of someone you care for and who cares for you. Picture them in front of you, perhaps returning your smile.

What are this person's good qualities? Why do you appreciate them? How have they helped you? Remember a kind or generous thing they did for you or for others.

The feeling of appreciation may increase. You can connect with them by wishing them happiness, health, safety—whatever words come to you: "I wish for you . . ."

Now consider what this person wishes for you. Do they wish for you to be free from pain and illness? To be happy? Imagine that you were hearing them from your friend or think about times they have told you directly. "I wish for you . . ."

Let yourself appreciate your friend's wishes for you. When you are ready, let go of the image of your friend and just rest in connecting with love and care. Notice how it feels in your body and in your heart.

It may take a few times of exploring this meditation before you genuinely connect with these feelings and wishes. That's okay, because even just going through the practice will begin to awaken the part of you that can connect with care for and from others. You can also try this practice with various people in your life.

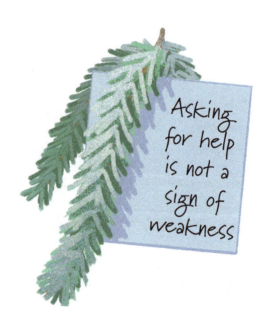

Asking for help is not a sign of weakness

From *How to Live Well with Chronic Pain and Illness*

by Toni Bernhard

Like many people, I always thought that asking for help was a sign of weakness and an imposition on others. Even after I became chronically ill and sometimes needed help badly, this attitude persisted. Then I had an experience that made me realize that asking for help can be an act of kindness toward others. Allowing them to help when you're struggling with your health makes them feel *less helpless* in the face of the new challenges in your life. It can mean a lot to someone to be able to aid a friend or family member who is struggling with his or her health. . .

And so I think it would be beneficial for we who are chronically ill to develop some skill at asking for help. We often need it, and most of those who care about us want to give it. I say "most" because every relationship is different. There may be people in your life who've never learned the joy of helping others. It's sad for them, and yet that's the way it is. In that case, think of other people to ask.

It takes practice to learn to ask for help. Most of us have to overcome a lifetime of conditioning in which we've been taught that only the weak need help. As a result, we cling to the notion "I can do everything myself," even though it may no longer be the case. . .

Think of your request as a gift from you: it gives this person a way to not feel helpless in the face of your health challenges. If you strike out, take a deep breath and try again. Even multi-million dollar baseball players get more than one strike!

A Forest of Care

Ming's Story

Asking for help has been really great. I have an excessive love of independence, and I don't like asking for help, but there's so much goodwill out there. I'll put something on Facebook like, "Is anyone going to my neighborhood in the next few days? I need help with something." And immediately, within fifteen or twenty minutes, somebody has seen it and writes, "I'm on my way."

If you just sit in your corner and suffer and never ask for help, then you'll be missing one of the most wonderful aspects of being so fucking sick, which is that there is just a huge web of goodwill out there, including from strangers. There's a wonderful, blooming forest of care that's invisible normally, and if you are super sick, then it lowers the barriers that are normally there. And I think if you keep those barriers up yourself by not asking or by not sharing where you are, then you're really depriving yourself of something wonderful.

From A.H. Reaume in *Disability Visibility: First-Person Stories from the Twenty-First Century*

There is so much that able-bodied people could learn from the wisdom that often comes with disability. But space needs to be made. Hands need to reach out. People need to be lifted up.

The story of disabled success has never been a story about one solitary disabled person overcoming limitations—despite the fact that's the narrative we so often read in the media. The narrative trajectory of a disabled person's life is necessarily webbed. We are often only as strong as our friends and family make us, only as strong as our community, only as strong as the resources and privileges we have.

Did you ask for help this week, even in a very small way?

Give yourself a gold leaf!

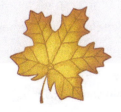

111

Mind, Body, Spirit Connection

Gloria's Story

I am an older, late-blooming lesbian. I was married and raised four children before I came out to myself. I identify a lot with my Hispanic background, which is from my dad. However, I was brought up in white culture. I have arthritis and fibromyalgia, and I eventually had to retire as a massage therapist due to my health. I'm now a spiritual director, which is a continuation of the mind/body/spirit connection that I learned initially through doing bodywork.

I was diagnosed with fibromyalgia in 1987, which was a new kind of diagnosis then, and there were a lot of doctors that did not believe my diagnosis at all. I had doctors say in front of me, "Well, that's a garbage diagnosis." One of the ways I've found support and connection is through bodywork and regular psychological therapy with people who understand chronic illness.

Chronic illness leads to isolation, and sometimes we can isolate ourselves without even knowing it. Years and years ago, when my family was very young, the stores in downtown Chicago used to have all of these beautiful window displays for Christmas. It was lovely. My husband at the time wanted to go down and see the displays with a small social group. I really didn't want to do that. I can't remember if I had a sore ankle or something, but some people lent us a wheelchair and I was pushed around in it. And I thought, "Oh, these windows are really beautiful. I'm really enjoying this."

I have said no to things that lead to isolation from my friends, from a new activity. I might want to go to see a new play and think,

"No, my back isn't feeling well enough to do that today. I don't want to sit in that uncomfortable chair." So it has a significant impact on my relationships with family, with my friends, and with church people. If I think about going to the symphony, I worry, "Oh no, those chairs are too squeezed in, this is not comfortable. I'm afraid to walk up to the balcony in case I fall down those stairs." I miss out on those connections, and sometimes I have to do that. I've learned over the years to say yes to what I *can* do, and to work with my body.

Recently, on a vacation with my wife, I used a walking stick to help keep myself steady while walking. It's interesting being this age ... I thought I was in touch with my body after all these years of massage therapy work. But now that I'm receiving regular bodywork again, those connections between body, mind, and spirit are coming back to me even more strongly, and they're making whatever discomfort that I have been feeling a little easier to deal with again.

Having chronic illness informs my practice as a spiritual director, knowing that the person I'm sitting across from may be going through something similar. Sometimes my clients are dealing with the same kind of frustrations about when things don't work out or when doctors don't believe them.

Ultimately, I believe that we need to pay more attention to Spirit. Despite the pain and aggravation, Spirit is back there someplace. If we can bring Spirit to the forefront, that can be a magnificent help for all the pain and frustration.

Journal Prompts

Isolation and Connection

To allow ourselves to feel fully alone is to allow ourselves to understand the particular nature of our solitary incarnation, to make aloneness a friend is to apprentice ourselves to the foundation from which we make our invitation to others.

DAVID WHYTE, *CONSOLATIONS*

- How has isolation shown up in your life? In relation to chronic illness or pain?

- Have you found ways to make aloneness a friend?

- How has connection shown up in your life? How does it show up now?

- What is one small step toward greater connection, if this is something you long for?

How Does Connection Show Up for Me?

by Mary Elizabeth White

I am soothed, calmed, and restored by seeing the moon moving across varied skies as she—sometimes orange—sometimes soft pastel—waxes and wanes. I am connected.

I am refreshed and reassured by reading poetry, absorbing images that extract me from ponderous thought and propel me vividly into the natural world. I am connected.

Crows and ravens cawing, calling early and late. The indescribable sound of flight and glimpses of their silent movement across gray skies. I am connected.

Moisture gathered on windowsills, dripping softly. Sunlight warming my skin. Awakening an unsuspected, forgotten optimism. The salty edge on ocean air in early mornings. I am connected.

How does connection show up?

When I see someone fight their own small self to become a conduit of compassion for another. When I see someone daring to believe that they are loved by another . . .

I am connected.

Reflection Questions

Isolation and Connection

- What did you learn from your family and culture about how your connections and relationships should be?

- What did you learn from your family or culture about asking for help or being dependent?

- How does chronic illness or pain affect your relationships and connections with community?

- If you long for more human connection, can you name those longings with compassion toward yourself?

- Are there ways you find connection that are not about other humans? In nature? In spirituality? With animals? With creativity?

Playlist for Isolation and Connection

Are You Lonesome Tonight? by Roy Turk and Lou Handman, sung by Elvis Presley

Lone Wolf by Lea Morris

Nobody Knows by Pink

All Will Be Well by Meg Barnhouse

Lean on Me by Bill Withers

Room at the Table by Carrie Newcomer

Stand by Me by Ben E. King, sung by Playing for Change

Crowded Table by the Highwaywomen

We Are by Sweet Honey in the Rock

Nobody Knows the Trouble I've Seen by Louis Armstrong, sung by Mahalia Jackson

Everybody Eats When They Come to My House by Cab Calloway

Breezy Slide by Louie Zong and Brian David Gilbert

7

Strength and Fortitude

If opening your eyes, or getting out of bed, or holding

a spoon, or combing your hair is the daunting

Mount Everest you climb today, that is okay.

Carmen Ambrosio

Winter can feel like a test sometimes. Did you put on the right coat? Can you get through the icy streets or make it up that hill? Winter takes fortitude, preparation, and planning. In ancient times, and for some even today, it can be a test of strength to survive the cold temperatures and food scarcity.

In Norse mythology, winter symbolizes the difficulty of life. Yule, a festival celebrating the sun's rebirth, occurs during this season. It is a reminder that we can get through the hard winters and that light returns. The winter solstice is an important reminder in religions across the world that days will once again grow longer and that you have made it through the deepest dark.

When temperatures drop, it can be a shock to the system. Winter can be a particularly difficult time for those living with chronic illness, sometimes triggering increases in discomfort and pain. Some illnesses and conditions can make you more susceptible to changes in weather and temperature. Emotional or physical stress during this darker season also can increase susceptibility to flares.

Getting through the winter while struggling with pain and chronic illness requires drawing on many external and internal resources. French philosopher Albert Camus, who suffered from tuberculosis and its aftereffects, wrote, "In the depth of winter, I finally learned that there was in me an invincible summer." This chapter will explore tools and approaches to find strength and fortitude when you need it the most.

When you hear the term *strength*, perhaps you first imagine someone physically strong. Or maybe you see it as the ability to power through challenges. Yet there are so many ways to view strength. One of the most important tools for people living with chronic health issues is to nurture emotional and spiritual resilience. Having more resilience in these areas helps with dealing with the roller coaster of unpredictable health. The inner reserves that are drawn on in the midst of recovery from surgery or debilitating pain are different for each person. What strength do you need in your life right now? How do you celebrate the strength and resilience you already have within you?

Strength Is More Than Spinach

Julianne's Story

> The greatest glory in living lies not in never falling,
> but in rising every time we fall.
>
> NELSON MANDELA

Living through upper Wisconsin winters for the past fourteen years has taught me a bit about strength and fortitude, both emotionally and physically. Getting outside on cold, dark mornings to clear my car of ice and snow has often felt like a herculean effort. In the South we only had to clear off pollen from our windshields, and only a rare bit of ice! My Southern-born children would wail about having to help shovel the drive and complain about the biting wind as we prepared for school each day. I thought getting them ready for elementary school with their snowsuits, scarves, and boots was enough of a challenge. Dealing with harsh winter temperatures in the grips of a flare is much more formidable.

When I was young, I had a mental picture of what strength looked like. I didn't have a magic lasso like Wonder Woman, but when I watched Popeye, I was convinced that if I ate enough spinach, I could grow strong like him. He could handle all of the bad guys, and everything turned out just fine at the end of each episode. I really wanted that too. As the youngest in my family, being strong was a good way to keep up with the older kids and hold my own in a fight with siblings. After watching one episode, I once asked my mom to make me spinach. I tried it a few different ways, but it was pretty yucky to my little taste buds. If I didn't like spinach, how else could I be strong?

Strength equaled safety to me when I was a little girl. I had a chaotic childhood in my kindergarten and elementary years, and physical strength made me feel more secure. I adored building forts, playing kickball and hide and seek, and biking through my neighborhood and the woods behind our house. I'd wrestle my best friend Brian and tried to be strong enough to climb the highest trees and bike farther than all the other kids

As we get older, many of us start to ask ourselves what strength means to us. Getting diagnosed with rheumatoid arthritis in my forties caused me to ask the same question again. I was frustrated with the unpredictability of my body and this disease. How would I handle days when it hurt to do basic tasks like using a stapler or taking a walk? Thankfully, those days don't happen often, though on some days I'm simply not able to do what I used to do. I've had to reframe my idea of what being strong looks and feels like. It has taken a big mental shift to let go of what I thought should happen and to accept the reality that I live in.

We all have our own story and have to figure out how to manage our struggles. Living with pain has caused me to develop a resolve and resilience that I didn't have before, just from the sheer effort it takes to get up and get things done on rough mornings. I've drawn on that resolve when I've made it through vital events when I would rather have been in bed hiding under the covers. And I've also come to understand that being strong is also admitting when I need to ask for help. Western culture valorizes self-sufficiency and endurance. That isn't a healthy mindset for anyone: all of us need support of one kind or another. You can move through that sense of vulnerability and fear of judgment to embrace that asking for help is a sign of courage and even wisdom.

There are so many ways to look at strength. Learning your limitations is also a source of strength. I will often start a walk with ambitions to go on the longer route around my neighborhood only to have to move to the shorter one due to pain. I've tried to shift my mindset from thinking of this as failure: it is honoring my body and where I am at that day. Being real with myself helps me take care of myself better; I'm less likely to get injured or try to do more than my body will allow.

Basketball coach John Wooden said, "Never let the things you cannot do prevent you from doing the things you can." I now ask my partner or children to help with heavy groceries or full laundry baskets. I try to do everything I can and acknowledge where I can't. And despite the frustration that brings sometimes, I know that I'm stronger by not pushing my body in unhealthy ways. Ultimately, we are stronger together—surrounded by community and support so that we need not do it alone.

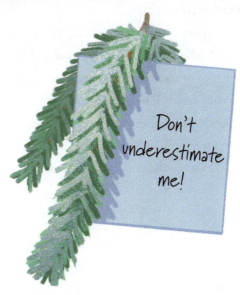

Don't underestimate me!

From "To Survive Climate Catastrophe, Look to Queer and Disabled Folks"

by Patty Berne, as told to Vanessa Raditz in *Disability Visibility: First-Person Stories from the Twenty-First Century*

In order to value others, we have to know our own worth. In this historical moment, we have to fight for the valuable lives of butterflies and moss and elders. Because our lives—and all life—depend on this. We must move beyond our cultural beliefs that tell us we are worth only as much as we can produce. Just as each component in Earth's ecosystem plays a vital role in supporting everything around it, so do each of us have an essential role to play in sustaining our communities, our environment, our planet.

In this time, people need strength models. Strength isn't just about momentary power to jump building to building; it is also the endurance to handle what is less than ideal. It's the gritty persistence that disabled people embody every day.

Even in the moments when we're in pain, when we're uncomfortable, when the task ahead feels overwhelming and we feel defeated by the sheer scope of everything that's wrong in the world, we don't have to give up on life or on humanity. Queer and trans disabled people know that, because that's how we live. At this moment of climate chaos, we're saying: Welcome to our world. We have some things to teach you if you'll listen so that we can all survive.

Spiritual Practice

Strength

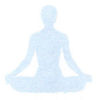

You have power over your mind—not outside events. Realize this, and you will find strength.

MARCUS AURELIUS

Not all strength comes from physical strength: building resilience can also be done on the inside. It can involve relating to what is sacred, finding meaning in daily and long-term tasks, or aligning with a cause or idea beyond oneself. This spiritual practice will assist you in identifying times you have felt strong and encourage you to build on those experiences.

For this spiritual practice, you are invited to set aside at least ten minutes. Pick a time when you can schedule quiet time to focus and be present in the practice.

Find a comfortable position and let your body relax. Try to breathe more slowly and deeply, giving yourself permission to be present to this moment.

Soften your gaze or close your eyes and imagine times when you have felt strength, whether spiritually, physically, or emotionally. How did that make you feel? What did that strength entail? What emotions or outcomes do you associate with it?

Try to remember and visualize other times you have felt strong. Was this on your own or with others? Pay attention to how your body and feelings respond when you imagine that sense of strength.

This practice can be repeated on a regular basis to build up your connection to strength in your life.

> Life's challenges are not supposed to paralyze you;
> they're supposed to help you discover who you are.
>
> BERNICE JOHNSON REAGON

We Parent Ourselves

Eric's Story

I'm a 69-year-old gay man in a long-term committed relationship. I've had a difficult life, and I have multiple medical issues. The longest is chronic depression, which I've had since I was six years old; the next longest is HIV, which I've had for 41 years; and the most recent is multiple myeloma (a cancer of the white blood cells), which I've had for 17 years.

Multiple myeloma used to have a 5% survival rate, but I got it just late enough that treatments have made it a chronically manageable illness, with long-term chemotherapy. Unfortunately, HIV and multiple myeloma affect two-thirds of my immune system. One hits the T cells, and the other hits the cells that produce antibodies.

Multiple myeloma can cause your entire bone structure to resemble having severe osteoporosis. My diagnosis occurred after the second vertebra in my neck just dissolved. There's a one in 2,000 chance of surviving that break, but I had no idea that I was near death. I was strong enough then that I was able to hold my head in place, walk into the bedroom, and lie down. I spent a month in the hospital afterward.

There have been times when my bones were so brittle that I would roll over in my sleep and crack a rib. At one point I was on a fentanyl patch and using an oxygen concentrator so I could breathe as shallowly as possible because it hurt so much just to breathe. It took everything I could to not panic, but by staying in a hypnotic state and having concentrated oxygen, I got through it.

Where have I found the strength to go on? Well, not having any alternatives is a tremendous tool for clearing and focusing the mind! And when I was studying psychology, I realized that as adults, we parent ourselves. I decided that if I was going to parent myself for the rest of my life, I needed to become the ideal, loving parent I needed when I was a child. If I had had someone like that in my earlier life, it would've been a lot less lonely. It is really one of the best pieces of advice I can give anybody. Be intentional about the way you parent yourself. It can get you through a lot.

Knowing self-hypnosis has made it possible for me to manage long-term pain much more effectively than I would otherwise. It's like having a little toolbox that can raise my endorphin levels and reduce my pain levels. It makes me feel calmer and more relaxed, so I can focus on what's important. And if I add some positive suggestions, like that I can get through this, that's even better. Because its benefits are so subtle, it can be hard to remind myself to do, but it helps me have that peace when I need it. I would recommend learning self-hypnosis for anyone in pain. You may not be able to just wish away what is hurting you, but you can take the most active, effective control you can when you're in that quiet, meditative state. It's almost as good as getting a good hug from someone who really cares about you.

And hugs are important. Also cats. On bad days, feeling that purr when one of my cats lies on my chest has a remarkably healing effect.

Having It Together

by Sarah York in *Into the Wilderness*

In my first year of ministry I received a request from a colleague that I lead a workshop for ministers on time management. My immediate response was, "You've got to be kidding! Me do a workshop on time management? You're talking to someone who puts in fifteen hours on a sermon between noon Saturday and 11:00 am Sunday—*after* I've done the research."

I said no to doing the workshop, but for the wrong reason. I thought I should have it together before presuming to speak to colleagues. Then I realized that if I waited until I had it together before I ever preached a sermon topic, we would be doing a lot of hymns and responsive readings on Sunday mornings.

It's a common misconception that strong people have it together and help those who aren't so strong. But how many people do you know who are so together that they don't need to reach out for help? If you know anyone like that, you probably don't like them very much. If they don't have any weaknesses, they can't understand yours very well.

And understanding is what we want from each other. Strength emerges when we know our own weakness. This is nothing new. But it doesn't hurt to remind ourselves from time to time that it's alright to be human.

Badass Warriors Among Us

by Tandi Rogers

I'm at the airport, tucked into a corner quietly working before my plane takes off in a couple hours. Through my headset I can hear more tone than words of a young woman a couple tables over from me. Her voice is measured and strong. She's taking someone to task but does not sound unkind. Then the phrase, "I am right here!" comes through my noise canceling device.

Moving my ear covering, I glance over. She's adamantly talking into her headset, saying things like, "I am calling about the care I'm receiving." "This is unacceptable!" "I have a right to this information. It is about me!" And "You can talk to me now or with my parents at my funeral. . ." Her voice is fierce and without apology.

I rip out a piece of paper and scrawl this note to her:

You are a fucking badass. I live with chronic illnesses that remain a mystery to doctors and I wish I had your presence and fierceness. Every time you advocate for yourself you help all of us. Bless you.

At first she looks confused as I slip this onto her table and respectfully back away. She reads it and we lock eyes, sending hand-hearts back and forth to each other. I start to cry, bow my head and pray for her safety and well-being. And for gratitude for her model of fierceness. I will remember her next time I am on the phone faced with medical erasure or gaslighting and try to conjure her strength and boldness.

Assignment

by Robert R. Walsh in *Noisy Stones*

While I am away, here are some things I want you to do. I want you to take care of yourself. Button up your overcoat. Fasten your seat belt. Eat your vegetables.

I want you to take care of someone else. Look for ways to help. Say, "I love you" (if you do). Hug a friend.

I want you to take care of your soul. Keep the different parts of yourself in touch with one another. Listen for quiet clues about the path your life should be following. Be aware of what kind of world you are helping to make each day.

Take good care.

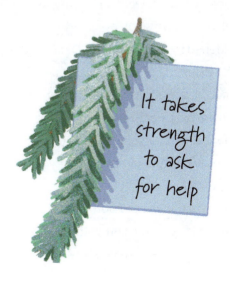

It takes strength to ask for help

Journal Prompts
Fortitude

In this journaling exercise, you're invited to imagine inspirations of strength that have held you in difficult times.

In *Loving Our Own Bones,* author Julia Watts Belser reflects on her fight to define her own path with strength, self-love, and fortitude:

> When I first came into the disability community, when I first began building the politics and relationships that would anchor me through the decades, it felt crucial to root my own identity in that bold refusal of healing and cure. I was emboldened by the example of Deaf activists, who fight for the recognition and protection of signing-Deaf cultures, even as technology and treatment offer increasing entry into the hearing world. My experience, of course, was not the same. I tried therapies and remedies, but everything cost more than it gained.
>
> And when it yielded nothing? I turned away. I said no to all the earnest empathy and to the world of pining. I could have stayed forever in the land of

wanting. Instead, I built a fierce and tender bedrock of radical self-love.

- What people or tools have helped you cope and find strength in the midst of chronic illness?

- Has self-love and acceptance of disability or illness helped support you in difficult times?

- How does it make you feel to read, "I love this body as she is, right here and now, with no regrets?"

- What words of love and encouragement would you give yourself or another?

Are you noticing the moments when you feel strong in your body, mind, or spirit? Are you connecting with health providers, friends, or family when you need outside support? Strength is knowing that you are not alone in your struggles; we all do better with support and connections. Kudos for taking care of yourself!

Give yourself a gold leaf!

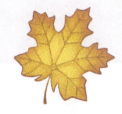

Reflection Questions
Strength

- What did your family, friends, or faith tradition teach you about what it meant to be strong while you were growing up? Were you given helpful tools to think about how strength can also be vulnerability or more than simply physical strength?

- How has the way you think about your own strength and others' changed or remained the same over time?

- What are your personal strengths? These can include traits such as compassion, leadership, resilience, and creativity.

- Strength is more than powering through difficult situations. Sometimes the biggest strength you can have is to understand when you need help. When have you relied on your own strength? When have you benefited from trusting others, relying on the strength of community and friends?

Playlist for Strength

Don't Ever Let Nobody Drag Your Spirit Down
by Eric Bibb

You Can Do This Hard Thing, by Carrie Newcomer

Rise Up by Andra Day

Choose Your Fighter by Ava Max

This Is Me by Benj Pasek and Justin Paul, sung by Keala
Settle and the cast of The Greatest Showman

Feelin' Stronger Every Day by Chicago

Anything Can Happen by Tors

Brave by Sara Bareilles

Fight Song by Rachel Platten

Warrior by Hannah Kerr

You Gotta Be by Des'ree

Up! by Shania Twain

Courage to Change by Sia

She Is a Warrior by Alita

Strength, Courage and Wisdom by India.Arie

I Didn't Know My Own Strength by Whitney Houston

8

Comfort

*You only have to let the soft animal of
your body love what it loves.*

Mary Oliver

During the long nights of winter, when we may feel that winter will last forever, it is good to have practices that can feed the body and the heart. Surely that is one of the reasons for the many festivals of light that happen in the winter, and for gathering and breaking bread together with beloved ones.

The winter of chronic illness or pain is also a time to develop practices that can feed the body and the heart. Finding comfort and pleasure can be a powerful way of working with pain and suffering, as the Zen teacher Darlene Cohen reminds us: "Among the most important healing experiences we can have are experiences of deep pleasure."

I have a sticky note on the door to my kitchen that reads, "How can I care for myself today?" It reminds me of my tender commitment to care for myself, physically, emotionally, and spiritually, as an essential part—perhaps the most essential part—of my healing journey toward living well, whatever my medical diagnoses and challenges. Friends and family can remind us to take care of ourselves and enjoy our lives, but we are responsible for actually doing so.

Finding pleasure, comfort, and ease in the simple things around us can make this hard season just a little bit easier, whether we are living through the literal season of winter or the winter within.

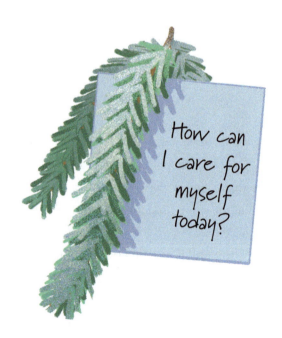

How can I care for myself today?

Spell for Rest and Renewal

by Atena O. Danner

I draw on the power of houseplants, candlelight, laughter, and dreaming to reclaim the rest that will heal me. In defiance of white supremacy, ableism, and patriarchy, I refuse to light the other end of my candle. I will boldly protect my softness, defend my sleep, and liberate all of my unassigned minutes, hours, and days. I am one soft animal among many: a cell in the breathing world's body. Let us be cared for as such. May it be so.

Hygge First Aid

Florence's Story

Early December a few years ago was rough. I had what I refer to as a snowball of medication complications, along with problems with doctors and seemingly endless bureaucratic struggles with insurance companies. The weather in Central Illinois was unremittingly dank and gray, to the point that a local meteorologist joked, on a rare sunny morning, that we might not immediately recognize that "bright light on the eastern horizon."

As a person who is immunocompromised due to medication, Covid isolation hadn't ended for me, and I live alone. I could feel myself sinking into sadness, loneliness, and joylessness. As a minister I am aware that midwinter is notorious for its emotional difficulty, but I'd never been hit quite so hard. What to do? I was in dire need of emotional first aid. Then I remembered hygge.

Hygge (pronounced, according to my Norse friends, HEW-guh) is a nearly untranslatable Scandinavian term meaning, among other things, comfort, coziness, connection, and contentment. It is not just a word but a way of life that has developed during the long, dark, challenging Scandinavian winters. Fires and candles are an essential part of hygge, as are friends, homemade food, and comfortable socks and blankets. Hygge is not about buying anything, but instead being grateful and connected to the simplest things.

That winter evening, I embarked on my hyggelig (yes, that's a word) makeover. Even though I knew I wouldn't be having friends over, I cleaned up my house as if friends *would* be coming over, but just for me. I found candles here and there and brought them all into the living room. I lit a fire in the wood stove and pulled a chair up in front of it. I made myself ginger snap cookies—and I'm not even a baker! I put on my comfiest socks and tuned the radio to classical Christmas music. I sat in the chair in front of the wood stove with a blanket around me, a book in my hand and a cat on my lap, munching on cookies I had made myself. Miraculously, I was already feeling better.

The next evening, I went out to an outdoor German-style Christmas market hosted by a local brewery. It was a little odd to go alone, but I pushed myself out the door as part of my first aid plan. I drank mulled wine from a paper cup and wandered past the little craft booths, feeling a bit at sea among all the happy families, then drifted toward a bonfire. I made a connection with a retired prairie biologist who was adding wood to the fire, and we happily chatted about goldenrod and native plants. By the time I came home I felt transformed.

All through the rest of December I baked—sharing my bounty with neighbors—lit candles, and made sure to enjoy the hauntingly beautiful choral music of the season. When the weather turned frigid, I kept the woodstove going night and day—much to the joy of my two cats, who were having their own hygge experience. I bought a small tree and set it up, with lights, right outside my front window, and noticed the intense pleasure I had every time I glanced at it. I cared for myself as an honored guest, and I was able to host my 94-year-old mother for Christmas, making a full Christmas meal for the first time in years. Somewhere along the way, I realized that my hard, sad mood had shifted to something gentler, kinder to myself, and comforted.

Spiritual Practice

Putting Comfort at the Top of the To-Do List

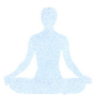

We have a tendency to think in terms of doing and not in terms of being. We think that when we are not doing anything, we are wasting our time. But that is not true. Our time is first of all for us to be. To be what? To be alive, to be peaceful, to be joyful, to be loving. And that is what the world needs most.

THICH NHAT HANH

We are human beings, not human doings, but our society tells us that productivity is one of the highest values of a human life. Many of us who are chronically ill are also very responsible: we are trying to hold down a job, take care of a family, and keep the house clean on top of getting to doctor's appointments, taking medications, eating well, and doing whatever else we need to do to stay afloat. The stress of *doing* can exacerbate our physical challenges. And in all that activity, finding ease and comfort can be far, far down the to-do list.

For this practice, you are invited to bring ease and comfort to the top of your to-do list.

Plan a brief vacation, just for you. This vacation could be as short as half an hour or as long as a day—you get to decide. Think of this time as a "comfort vacation."

What would you do if comfort and pleasure were at the top of your to-do list? Would you curl up in a soft blanket and read that book you've been wanting to read? Would you lie in the sun like an old cat? Would you listen to a guided meditation or play one of the songs on the Comfort playlist and let it wash over you? Would you get a massage? Would you take a cup of tea into the garden?

Now that you've planned your vacation, find a way to do it. This is your time—spend it in exactly the way that will give you the most pleasure. (Although a word of advice: we suggest choosing an activity that is *not* mindlessly scrolling on your phone or laptop!)

Or you can continue the spiritual practice from the Pain chapter of finding comfort and pleasure right where you are, right now, and savoring it.

Try this as often as you can.

Have you done something really nurturing for yourself today, like you would for a good friend?

Give yourself a gold leaf!

Stress, Hoodies, and a Good Cat

Valerie's Story

I am an African American woman in my sixties. My family moved to the South when I was nine, and there was intense racial prejudice there. While I experienced a lot of love from my mother, there was also strife between my parents. I was a social worker for many years, though I am currently in seminary and training to become a chaplain. I have considered myself a feminist since I was about twelve years old, and I practice both Buddhism and some forms of Catholicism. I consider myself a thinking Catholic.

When I was in my thirties, I was a social worker in a very high stress job, and I began to have digestive problems. It took a while for me to realize that I should go to a doctor, where I was diagnosed with irritable bowel syndrome (IBS). After beginning treatment, it was better, but every time there was extra stress in my life, it would become exacerbated. Now I recognize that even if I think if I'm dealing with a stressful event just fine, my body registers it in a different way, usually a day or two later.

A few years later when I was working for a large children's hospital, I was in a meeting with all the social workers in the hospital—about fifty of us—and we began talking about our health challenges. The number in the room who said they too had some form of somatic illness was stunning to me. I had always thought of my illness as *my* problem, my inability to deal with stresses, not as something that was part of the profession of social work, a result of working in a high stress profession. That really changed how I saw it, and myself. And being a Black woman

—well, as Black people we face day-to-day high stress all the time in this society, and that cuts across all socioeconomic lines.

Around that same time, I started having trouble with my vision. Again I downplayed it, though I finally went to the hospital. They misdiagnosed me initially, and I had to stand up for myself with the doctors, but eventually I was seen by a rheumatologist and diagnosed with sarcoidosis, an autoimmune inflammatory disease that can affect many parts of the body. It manifested in my lungs, my eyes, and my ears, affecting my hearing. I was on prednisone and methotrexate for about a decade and had problems with chronic sinus infections during that time too.

Having chronic illness and fatigue means I have to sleep more than other people. Friends who have not faced long-term illness just don't understand, and sometimes take it personally if I need to cancel my plans because I have run out of energy. That's hard.

I do know what brings me comfort, though. You'll laugh, but I've just discovered hoodies in the last few months. They gave them to us in our chaplaincy program, and I had no idea they were so comfortable. I see why people wear them now! Wearing my hoodie makes me feel safe and cocooned, especially if my cat Oliver comes and curls up with me—he likes it too. Cats bring me a lot of comfort, both my own cat and those I cat-sit. I love to read. Napping is great. And I love to be outside in nature, though I don't do enough of that.

If I could offer one piece of advice to someone who is new to chronic illness, it would be to be kind to your body.

From "A Burst of Light: Living with Cancer"

by Audre Lorde in *A Burst of Light and Other Essays*

Coming in out of the D.C. winter storm felt like walking into an embrace. The roaring fireplace, the low-beamed wooden room filled with beautiful Black and Brown women, a table laden with delicious foods so obviously cooked with love. There was sweet potato pie, rice and red beans, black beans and rice, pigeon peas and rice, beans and pimentos, spaghetti with Swedish meatballs, codfish and ackee, spinach noodles with clam sauce, five-bean salad, fish salad, and other salads of different combinations....

I want to live the rest of my life, however long or short, with as much sweetness as I can decently manage, loving all the people I love, and doing as much as I can of the work I still have to do.

Sometimes I feel like I'm living on a different star from the one I am used to calling home. It has not been a steady progression. I had to examine, in my dreams as well as in my immune-function tests, the devastating effects of overextension. Overextending myself is not stretching myself. I had to accept how difficult it is to monitor the difference. Necessary for me as cutting down on sugar. Crucial. Physically. Psychically. Caring for myself is not a self-indulgence, it is self-preservation, and that is an act of political warfare.

Journal Prompts

Comfort

Pick one of these as a journaling exercise or explore all three.

- From where you are sitting or lying down, how many things can you see, hear, taste, touch, and smell that bring comfort? List them in your journal. Then spend some time savoring each one, noticing them more deeply. Pick three to write about: in what ways do they bring comfort? Are there ways you could bring these objects or experiences into more of your daily life? You could do this in various locations and rooms.

- What people in your life bring the most comfort to you, and why? List them in your journal. Consider how you could connect more with the people you named, and write those ways down too. Then choose at least one concrete action you will do in the next week to cultivate your connection with one of the people.

- What are some actions that bring comfort and pleasure to you? Being wrapped in blankets? Getting into a particular yoga pose? A good long hug? Stroking a pet? (They like this too!) Holding a cup of warm tea? List as many as you can think of. Choose three to do today, and then write about what it was like to consciously choose an action of comfort and pleasure.

Reflection Questions

Comfort

- Did you have family rituals that brought you pleasure and comfort as a child? Were they daily, weekly, seasonal?

- What is a time in your life when pleasure or comfort was very important and nourished you?

- What kind of comfort might you want to bring into your life that is not there now?

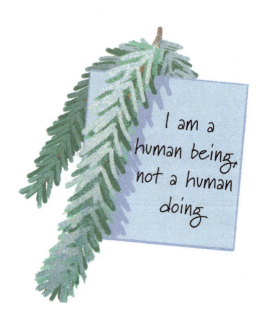

Playlist for Comfort and Peace

Comfort Me by Mimi Bornstein-Doble, sung by Linli Wang

Filled with Loving Kindness, adapted from Buddhist meditation by Mark Hayes, performed by Ian W. Riddell, Brian Kenny, and Alena Hemingway

Meditation on Breathing by Sarah Dan Jones, performed by the First Unitarian Society of Denver

Lean on Me by Bill Withers, sung by Lea Morris

We Need You by Cleo Sol

December by George Winston

Sending You Light by Melanie DeMore, performed with Julie Wolf

Sanctuary by Carrie Newcomer

Thula Thula (African lullaby), sung by Samite

Kothbiro (Rain Is Coming) by Ayub Ogada

Inner Peace by Beautiful Chorus

Lullaby for a Stormy Night by Vienna Teng

Spiegel im Spiegel by Arvo Pärt, performed by Leonhard Roczek and Herbert Schuch

Peace Be with Us by Ruth Cunningham, sung by Lea Morris

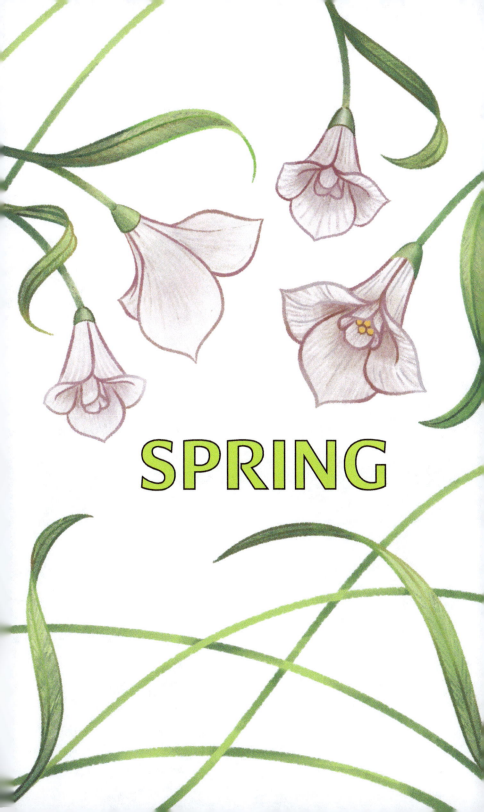

SPRING

SPRING

by Florence Caplow

As a child growing up in the Midwest, spring was my favorite season. I would watch eagerly for the day the grass turned green. It seemed to happen overnight: one day all the lawns around town would be straw-brown and matted from the snow, and then the next day I would wake up to emerald-colored lawns, like a magical transformation in the middle of the night. It was especially wonderful if the grass turned green on my birthday in early April; I superstitiously thought it meant I would have a particularly good year. I always wanted to spend my birthday outside in a park or in the woods, to celebrate the daffodils and early wildflowers shyly coming up through last year's dead leaves.

In my early teens, as I began to experience depression, spring became the hardest season. All that happy new growth contrasted sharply with the heavy winter in my heart. I felt out of step with the rest of the world and ashamed for not being in sync with the beauties of spring. Each year my depression would worsen in that season.

As a young adult, my discovery of meditation gradually led me out of depression, and spring became once again a time of joy. When I was in my early twenties I attended my first silent Buddhist meditation retreat, in Northern California. It was March, and the open grassy hills around the retreat center were clothed in shades of green of an intensity I had never seen before, which I later came to call hallucinatory green. The long hours of meditation practice opened my heart and my eyes, and I kept thinking of William Blake, who wrote, "If the doors of perception were cleansed everything would appear . . . as it is, infinite."

Later, as a working botanist in the Pacific Northwest, each spring I would head out into the shrub-steppe of eastern Washington in search of rare plants. I remember the feeling of driving east, crossing Snoqualmie Pass, and driving down from the mountains, until the forests opened up to great, green grassy hills filled with wildflowers. Every time, my heart would leap up in joy at those great open vistas after a winter in the soggy, tangled western part of the state. I knew I would spend the next few months walking under the sun, identifying and studying the plants we found. Spring was a time of freedom.

I no longer work in those hills. Chronic illness has brought its many limitations. But now I rejoice in my garden in the spring, full of flowers and shrubs I have planted over the years, finding joy where I can.

When I think of spring, one of the words that comes to mind is "tentative." Everywhere I have lived—the Pacific Northwest, California, the Rocky Mountains, the Midwest—spring, of all the seasons, is the most uncertain and unpredictable. When I lived in the Northwest, I had a Frost peach in my yard, bred for shorter growing seasons, and some years it flowered and bore many sweet fruits. But despite its name, other years a late frost would wither the flowers or the rains would be too unrelenting to allow the pollinators to fly, and there would be no peaches that year.

As a Midwestern gardener now, I notice that many of us get excited about spring long before it makes sense to start turning over the soil, and each year the people at the nurseries have to remind us that it's a bit too early, even if the sun is shining. Unless I am willing to plant pansies, which seem to be able to withstand anything, I need to practice patience until spring has fully committed to itself.

In the seasons of chronic illness and pain, spring can appear when there is hope or evidence of healing. Nonetheless, many of us live with conditions where unpredictability is a daily reality. Will I be able to weed my garden today, or is this a day where the body dictates rest? There is the all-too-common experience of one step forward in recovery and two (or more) steps back, which can be almost worse than never taking that step forward in the first place.

Spring is also a time, as I experienced as a teen, where the whole world seems to be celebrating, and shame can arise if the state of the body or the mind makes it impossible to join the celebration. Finally, we included a chapter on caregiving and self-care in this season, knowing that many people with chronic illness or pain are also caregivers for others. In fact, caregiving itself significantly increases the risk of developing chronic physical conditions and limitations.

In this section, you will find reflections, meditations, spiritual practices, stories and quotes on spring's gifts and challenges: hope and recovery, unpredictability, shame, and caregiving, and ways of practicing with them: connecting with kindness toward yourself, resting in not knowing, celebrating hope, and remembering self-care.

9

Hope

*Living with chronic illness isn't a life half-lived;
it's an opportunity to redefine what it means
to be truly alive, resilient, and whole.*

Christopher Reynolds

Hope is the unexpected gift, a verdant garden blooming in rocky soil. It is like learning something you thought was a weed is a beneficial herb, with a fragrant scent and many uses. In *Soil: The Story of a Black Mother's Garden,* Camile T. Dungy writes,

> That swamp milkweed didn't flower the 2017 summer my mother first noticed it, but years later, in 2020, the pink-petaled plant thrived among the hearty survivors crowded into the door yard. Hollyhocks; purple penstemon; white-petaled, yellow eyed Shasta daisies; upright prairie coneflowers; purplish-pink echinacea; and big red fireballs of bee balm like out of a sci-fi film about affable, non-Earth-dwelling sentient beings.

In spring we are reminded that out of the slumbering earth, life rises green and new again. Bulbs that have rested in the dark of winter emerge into the light of warmer days. Hope is much like that—when we need it the most, it can emerge from deep wells within us and bring new beginnings and beauty to our lives. Camile T. Dungy writes further,

> Finally mature, this cluster of plants grew in differently from what I imagined when I dug up rock beds and threw down seed. It takes three years for plants in a garden to achieve their potential, still longer to fully establish themselves. Working in this yard, I've learned a great deal about biding time, about accepting that change does not happen overnight and often shows up differently than I expect.

Hope can improve quality of life when living with chronic disease. Research has found that hope is associated with improved coping, well-being, and engagement in healthy behaviors in young adults. Among teens, hope is linked with health, quality of life, self-esteem, and a sense of purpose. It is an essential factor for developing both maturity and resilience. At any age, hope is a positive force in our lives. It can help us face what seems insurmountable or give us the strength to get through a painful day.

It is possible to have hope even with permanent health conditions. You might hope to have better pain control with a new medicine or hope to see more mobility with physical therapy. Hope can be as simple as noticing the beauty around you and letting it be a wind at your back.

In this chapter, you are invited to ponder threads of hope and recovery and explore these themes with journal prompts, spiritual practices, and music. How can you cultivate hope as a practice? What hope do you need right now?

When You Reach for Hope

Julianne's Story

> Hope is being able to see that there is light despite
> all of the darkness.
>
> DESMOND TUTU

I've always been someone who sees the glass half full instead of half empty. I think this helps me in my own pain management and coping skills with rheumatoid arthritis. It doesn't mean I'm living in denial; it means that I lean into a mental framework that points out the positives. This helps me through tougher days.

I have an important mentor, Sue, whom I've known for many years. She was diagnosed with rheumatoid arthritis early in life. Sue has had over thirty surgeries in the years that she's battled the disease, and I learned a lot from her example of living a full life. I saw how she leans into spiritual practices of joy, creativity, and centering to cope with her chronic pain. I saw that it wasn't easy for her to lean into hope, but it made her days more bearable.

Reaching for hope feels risky sometimes. We might get our hopes dashed when things don't turn out like we wanted. Where I live in Wisconsin, we endure the long, cold winters waiting for shoots of green to peek through the snow as a sign for long-awaited spring. Hope can feel like that, a ray of color or light when everything else feels forbidding.

Reaching for hope is also a bit like searching for the aurora borealis. Will it be cloudy? Can you stay up late enough to see them, and are you in the right location? I witnessed the haunting beauty of the aurora twice this year in Wisconsin. It was like I was in the presence of some cosmic dance or a mythical being. I'd spent many nights driving out to remote locations, checking my aurora app religiously for the times and places to look. It was frustrating to constantly miss them despite all of my attempts. When I finally was lucky enough to catch them, I knew it was something I'd always remember. Hope is the gumption to keep going, whether it is chasing good health outcomes or the right spot to catch the northern lights. You don't know if you'll be successful, but you feel as if you need to try.

I was twenty-six when my mother was diagnosed with stage four lung cancer, in 1999. My brother drove all the way from South Carolina to Atlanta to let me know. At first, I was in complete shock. I was also incredibly angry about how many times I'd asked her to stop smoking. Though I knew how hard it was to quit, it gave me something other than grief to focus on. I was going to lose my mom, and she'd never get a chance to see my future children. I wouldn't get to see her grow old.

Meanwhile, she had wild hopes for a miracle, for more time with her children and grandchildren, and she planned to attend my wedding in April of 2000. My hopes were more tempered: I hoped for treatments and medicine that could prolong her time with us. I was desperate for every good day and visit I could have with my mama.

She made it through our wedding shower and she kept promising she'd be at the wedding, even if she was there in the wind. She died two weeks before my wedding, but I swear she was there in the breeze that kept blowing out our unity candle at the ceremony. And some say they saw a butterfly at the edge of the clearing where we were married.

HOPE

Hope kept her alive for eighteen months past her diagnosis. She loved and fought hard, and so did her doctors. What I learned most of all about hope from my mother is that it doesn't mean that everything is fine. It means that there are places of light and love, and you can hold onto those good things and let them lift you.

Spiritual Practice

Hope

Taking care of yourself is an important spiritual practice. What are your support resources? Who do you talk with when you're struggling? In a troubled world, full of stressful headlines and worries about loved ones, it can be hard to feel optimistic. And yet hope has never been more desperately needed.

Below are two spiritual practices to help you strengthen your connection to hope and resilience.

- Start each day with messages that support you. If you find the firehose of news or social media stressful, there are other ways to begin your day. Podcasts on gratitude or meditation, hobby-focused websites or books, and Sudoku or other puzzles are a few options. There are also newsletters that focus on sharing good news.

- Each day, note three things that are beautiful, uplifting, or bring you hope. In our hardest times, it can be hard to see past the obstacles. Noting these things can help bring light and a larger perspective. You might choose to add them to a journal or put them on sticky notes where you can see them as a supportive reminder.

bare bones

by ullie-kaye

hope is not always soft and lovely.
she is not always cascading rivers
and sunlit skies, dancing. hope knows
there is work to be done. there are
roads to be traveled. turns to be made.
she is bare bones and deep waters.
she is weary and weak. she is barely
a glimmer. she shakes when she speaks.
this is where hope lives. smothered in
sweat. full of war. and on the verge
of crumbling into the sea.
yet there she is, quietly breathing.

*We all need time to heal and recover from hurts
both physical and emotional. Are you noticing
the moments when you need time to nurture your
body, mind, or spirit? Are you pausing to notice and
breathe when you are overwhelmed and need to
take a break?*

Give yourself a gold leaf!

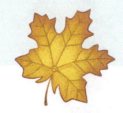

From *My Soul Showed Up: Finding Hope and Resilience Against All Odds*

by Pat Henneberry

When I have hope, I feel like I can take on the world. My pain might still be high, but with hopefulness on my side, I can banish—if only for a moment—the lies that anxiety and fear have been trying to sell me. With hope, there is a vision of a future where my back pain is manageable, and I can make plans for a new life. Instead of waking up with no blueprint at all, hope lets me dream of better days ahead. The steady stream of questions bouncing around in my mind is replaced with grace. When I have hope, it's like riding the easiest wave to shore. And like the ocean waves, hope ebbs and flows within me.

I've learned how fragile hope can be and how it needs to be nurtured to fight against the dark forces of fear. When you are filled with it, you want to hold on forever and savor every moment. Optimism can be fleeting, and sometimes if you try and grab it harder, it slips through your fingers. Thus, hope teaches us to live in the moment, not knowing when its warmth will shine again but ready to enjoy every moment of its healing powers. Hope often takes me by surprise. I can be having the worst day of physical pain when its vice grip eases ever so slightly. Suddenly, I'm able to take a deep breath or two, not even aware that I had been holding my breath to grit through the pain.

Moments of Joy

Bob's Story

I'm an older white gay man who lives with multiple chronic illnesses and will soon retire from being an English professor. I have long struggled with a mysterious form of digestive hypersensitivity. This hypersensitivity has been very difficult for doctors to understand and find ways to treat. I've also long struggled due to the impact of living with epilepsy. Most recently I was diagnosed with lupus. Like many who live with chronic illnesses, I don't always cope with these as well as I'd like.

Moments of joy can help. There are moments that can help me transcend the pain and hardship of the many difficult days I experience. Suddenly the sun will come out or a shy student will open up to share profound insights. My relationship with my husband Andy and our dog Aidan is a recurrent source of joy. Living with chronic illness for so long, I've learned to look for bright spots, even faint glimmers of hope, amid the darkest days. I have learned to show more compassion toward myself and especially others, but I still need to do a lot to improve with the former. Other people often don't recognize or understand what I'm going through, and that can make it especially difficult. I strive to keep in mind I don't know what they're experiencing either.

Recently, I've been learning about radical acceptance through acceptance and commitment therapy. It has helped me accept my health obstacles rather than feeling guilty or ashamed for not overcoming them. I have tried to accept what is out of my control, to recognize that I can't control my health all the time. So much in chronic illness fluctuates uncontrollably. To accept that it is the illnesses that are out of control and not me has been important. I try to feel at peace with where I am at and let go of worry concerning what I should be doing, although this is far from easy for me.

I need, most of all, to let go of being anxious that I'm anxious (generalized anxiety disorder is yet another chronic illness I deal with). I often reflect that I've dealt with many difficult challenges before and have gotten through them. I try to remember this when I'm having an especially tough time that I have been through difficult times before and made it through. It is helpful for me to reflect on what is going on and what has gone on with me, always very carefully attuned to my body, while countering counterproductive thought patterns when they arrive.

I have learned to be somewhat more patient as I've lived with chronic illness, with myself and especially with others, but this learning process is continually ongoing, just as is my experience of the impacts of living with chronic illness.

> At times our own light goes out and is rekindled by
> a spark from another person. Each of us has cause
> to think with deep gratitude of those who have
> lighted the flame within us.
>
> ALBERT SCHWEITZER

From *Beyond the Mailbox: A Life with Chronic Illness*

by Pat Gavula

"Just take it one day at a time." Well, how else am I supposed to take my life? Two days at a time? A week at a time? Sometimes I need to take life one hour at a time. With this illness it is impossible to look too far into the future since symptoms can change from morning to afternoon to evening. I have to take life as it presents itself.

"Have you tried (fill in the blank with a treatment you've heard of but may never have tried)." Trust me. I've tried everything within reason and a few options on the margins. I am done with that. I cannot get my hopes up once again and risk having them dashed. If someone had a definitive treatment I'd take it. Otherwise, it seems better to just cope with what I have. . . .

I know you are just trying to help and be kind but, please, no platitudes. Spend a day or a week in my body and then see what you'd like people to say to you. Perhaps something like this:

"I cannot imagine how you feel."

"I don't know if I could tolerate what you put up with all the time."

"I'm sorry this is happening to you."

"I wish I could take all this away."

"You don't deserve this."

"I don't know what to say."

"I wish I had the words/means to help you feel better."

"What would be most helpful for you today?"

"I love you and I care."

Thus It Was

by Dag Hammarskjöld

I am being driven forward
Into an unknown land.

The pass grows steeper
The air colder and sharper
A wind from my unknown goal
Stirs the strings of expectation.

Still the question
Shall I ever get there?
There where life resounds
A clear pure note in the silence.

From "Nurturing Black Disabled Joy"

by Keah Brown in *Disability Visibility:*
First-Person Stories from the Twenty-First Century

I may not find joy every day. Some days will just be hard, and I will simply exist, and that's okay, too. No one should have to be happy all the time—no one can be, with the ways in which life throws curveballs at us. On those days, it's important not to mourn the lack of joy but to remember how it feels, to remember that to feel at all is one of the greatest gifts we have in life. When that doesn't work, we can remind ourselves that the absence of joy isn't permanent; it's just the way life works sometimes. The reality of disability and joy means accepting that not every day is good but every day has openings for small pockets of joy.

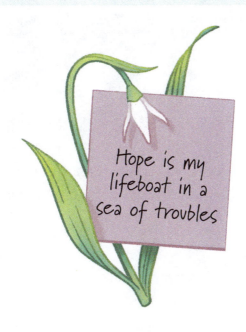

Hope is my lifeboat in a sea of troubles

Journal Prompts

Hope

Close your eyes and imagine a time when you experienced hope in your life. Think about other examples, if you can recall them, and list them in your journal with as much detail as you find helpful. Then spend some time with each one, noticing what emotions or thoughts arise.

Hope can be essential to get through each day when dealing with chronic illness, but with the unpredictability of health, hopes can also be unrealized and feel disheartening. What is the breadth of your experiences?

- What are some of your current hopes and dreams?

- Do your past experiences affect how you experience hope in the present?

- Choose one current hope or an experience in your past and work with it today. Notice any feelings or thoughts that arise and try to follow those cues.

Reflection Questions

Hope

As long as we have hope, we have direction, the energy to move, and the map to move by.

LAO TZU

- What did your family, friends, or beliefs teach you about hope?

- What are some of your experiences with hope making a difference in your life or in the life of someone that of you know?

- Are there hopes that you find easier to imagine than others?

- Is hope useful for you, or does it get in your way?

- What role does hope play in your life or in your wellness journey?

Playlist for Hope

Resilient by Rising Appalachia

Freedom by Jon Batiste

I'm Like a Bird by Nelly Furtado

Shake It Off by Taylor Swift

Pocketful of Sunshine by Natasha Bedingfield

Every Day by Rascal Flatts

You're Gonna Be OK by Brian and Jenn Johnson

I Was Here by Beyoncé

Underdog by Alicia Keys

A Drop of Water by Dana Lyons

10

Change and Unpredictability

The only way to make sense out of change is to plunge into it, move with it, and join the dance.

Alan Watts

"Unpredictable" could be spring's power word. Of all the seasons, spring seems to be the one with the most dramatic swings: one day balmy, the next sleeting. In the Midwest, spring is the season of tornadoes that can strike without warning, destroying everything in their path. But then the next day the sun may be shining and summer seems to be around the corner. It all depends on the day. So it is with many chronic conditions and especially autoimmune diseases, which tend to follow patterns of relapse and improvement. One day life can feel nearly normal, and the next day the symptoms are back, disabling as ever.

The uncertainty and unpredictability of many chronic illnesses mean any kind of planning ahead is difficult. This can be a source of bewilderment and grief for us and everyone around us when once again, for the umpteenth time, cherished plans need to be changed or cancelled. It also makes working a full-time job, with just a few days of sick leave available every year, next to impossible, with consequences for long-term financial stability. Those with GI illnesses sometimes can't even plan a few hours ahead.

The central teaching of Buddhism is that the nature of the universe is change and impermanence and the primary cause of suffering is our resistance to that fact. The Buddha taught that "Nothing is permanent except change." Those of us with chronic illness know this in our bones, though not without considerable misery and frustration. The question is: can we learn to dance with these changes? Can we learn to accept that not only do we experience unpredictability in our own bodies, but this is the nature of the universe itself? That we are not alone in having to adapt to change?

In Zen we talk about don't-know mind. A mind that is certain about what will happen next is a closed and limited mind. A mind that is open to being surprised is a fluid and expansive mind. There is also a secret advantage to change: yes, today might be miserable, but there is always the possibility that tomorrow may be a good day, maybe even a great one. And for some of us, there is even the possibility of long-term remission or fully regaining our health and well-being. And whether our bodies heal or not, it is possible to experience healing of the spirit.

This chapter explores the nature of unpredictability and offers support for the journey toward a life of adapting to the body's changes with grace.

At times I'm completely free of symptoms; at other times I lie in bed curled in a ball around the pain, and feel nausea so persistent that food—and life—loses all savor and joy. Every plan is subject to the body's unpredictability: tea with a friend, a hike in the mountains, a retreat with a favorite teacher—all may seem reasonable when first imagined, impossible when the time arrives. When the symptoms return, life becomes very small and narrow—the width of a bed, the space between one aching limb and another. And I feel grief. It's hard to hurt, again; it's hard to have to put one's life on hold, again; it's hard to be back in the place of illness. This is the territory of the dark fields.

FLORENCE CAPLOW, "DANCING IN THE DARK FIELDS"

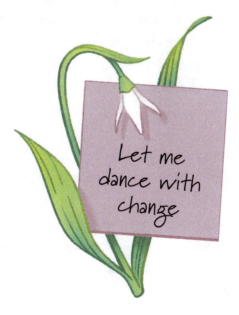

Let me
dance with
change

Comfortable with Uncertainty, Open to Contingency

Florence's Story

I was thirty-five years old when chronic illness first struck me, but I had no idea it was going to be chronic. Few healthy people can even imagine being chronically ill in their twenties or thirties. I made my living as a field biologist, which is intensely physical work, and I was used to being strong and capable. Almost overnight I was weak, nauseous, feverish, and in pain. Once I started to feel better, I assumed that the symptoms that had plagued me were now gone, thank God, and I could get on with my active life, my real life. I plunged back into all the things I loved to do.

And then the exact same set of symptoms came back, and my active life stopped all over again. And then I gradually got better. And then it came back. This pattern happened over and over again, like a repeated, discordant melody. Each time I got better I was sure that it was gone for good, and each time I was proved wrong. And I could never predict how long either state would last—it could be days, weeks, or months. For the first two years I didn't even have a diagnosis.

I often blamed myself when the symptoms recurred: I must have done too much, not gotten enough sleep, not eaten right—anything to explain why it was happening again. But the reality was that no matter what I did or didn't do, it came back. And each time it did, I would go through another round of grief, bewilderment, isolation, anger, uncertainty—the many faces of being chronically ill.

It took me two years of this yo-yo life to be diagnosed and to understand that this was the pattern of my particular form of chronic illness, undifferentiated connective tissue disease (UCTD). I had moved from the realm of the healthy to the realm of those with debilitating physical challenges. For twenty-five years I have been practicing acceptance of my various chronic illnesses. Now, with autoimmune rheumatoid arthritis, the stakes are higher and the possibilities more dire, but even with this disease I have times of being less symptomatic and times of more symptoms and more disability.

Shortly after my diagnosis with rheumatoid arthritis, my Zen teacher invited me to begin preparation for what is called, in my tradition, dharma transmission: full empowerment of a Soto Zen priest as an independent teacher, something that only happens after many years as a Zen student and ordained priest. Dharma transmission is a long and solemn process of preparation followed by an eight-day private ceremony. The Covid pandemic was raging and we were living in different regions of the country, so the study and preparation was via Zoom and on my own, but we both knew that at some point I would need to make it to his home in California from my home in Illinois for the ceremony itself.

Over the two years we were preparing for the ceremony, rheumatoid arthritis profoundly changed the shape of my life. I had to leave my work as the lead minister of a Unitarian Universalist congregation due to profound fatigue, and I went on long-term disability. The drugs I needed to take for my condition affected my immune system and the ability of my body to make antibodies to Covid, even with vaccines. My teacher, in his eighties, developed a rare autoimmune illness himself, and he became part of the population most vulnerable to Covid. How could I safely get to

California for the ceremony without catching Covid myself or bringing it to him?

Every time we tried to make plans, either my health or a surge in the pandemic made it impossible to travel. We started quoting the Buddhist teacher Pema Chodron to each other when we talked by Zoom, like a mantra: "Comfortable with uncertainty, comfortable with uncertainty." As Pema Chodron also wrote: "The truth is that things are always in transition. 'Nothing to hold on to' is the root of happiness. If we allow ourselves to rest here, we find that it is a tender, nonaggressive, open-ended state of affairs. This is where the path of fearlessness lies."

At least I had some experience with an unpredictable body: the autoimmune disease that I developed twenty years before had given me endless opportunities to develop patience and forbearance in the face of uncertainty. It's like riding waves: you just meet each wave as it comes.

We made plans and cancelled them, made plans and cancelled them. When I finally arrived at my teacher's house in western Sonoma County, he showed me the 800-year-old coast redwood on the property, and I thought of all the storms that redwood had endured, all the droughts, all the changes. And still it stood, hollowed out in the center by some fire, its feathery branches caressing the sky.

On the second day of our eight-day ceremony, my teacher injured his back and was immediately plunged into overwhelming pain. Suddenly we were back asking ourselves, "Can we be comfortable with uncertainty?" There was no knowing if he would be able to continue with the ceremony. With immense effort, and on strong pain medication, he continued. A few days later, I was on a walk down the dirt road that ran to the house, and

I found an enormous maple leaf in the middle of the road. I picked it up and brought it back, found ink and a brush, and wrote on it: "Comfortable with uncertainty; Open to contingency," and placed it on the altar.

Miraculously, given all the many challenges, we completed the ceremonies. The last ceremony takes place at midnight, and afterward we walked out into the fields below the house, in our formal Zen robes, the stars bright above us, great silence all around. He had told me stories of the mountain lion that had been seen nearby, and we heard some rustling from the edge of the field. It could have been anything—deer, raccoon, or the lion. And still we stood, breathing in the night air, not knowing what came next.

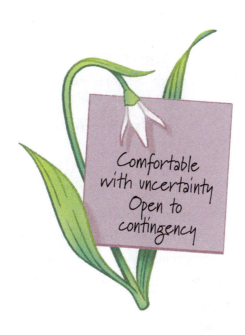

Spiritual Practice

Exploring Change

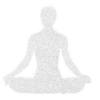

Things falling apart is a kind of testing and also a kind of healing. We think that the point is to pass the test or to overcome the problem, but the truth is that things don't really get solved. They come together and they fall apart. Then they come together again and fall apart again. It's just like that. The healing comes from letting there be room for all of this to happen: room for grief, for relief, for misery, for joy.

PEMA CHODRON, *WHEN THINGS FALL APART*

Here are three practices for exploring change.

- Find a lovely place outside with a comfortable place to sit. Set a timer for fifteen minutes and see how many changes you notice in that time, keeping your eyes open. Did birds fly overhead or start to sing? Did leaves move in the wind? Did the sound of a car get louder and then disappear? Did an ant crawl by? Were there changes in your own body: blinking, sighing, shifting position? How about in your mind: did you get restless, peaceful, start thinking about something? You may be amazed at just how much happens in fifteen minutes.

- Sit inside and put on a favorite piece of music, in any style. For this practice, please close your eyes and listen closely. Notice whether the music gets louder or softer, how the melody appears and disappears, and if the melody repeats or new voices or instruments appear. Consider that without change, there would be no music.

- Keep track of the changes in your body for three days. If you can, three times a day at the same time (setting a timer helps with this), note what is happening in your body and how you feel, writing down a brief description. Notice how differently you feel at various times, even a few hours apart.

The Farmer's Son

A Traditional Chinese Taoist story

An old farmer had a horse that broke loose and disappeared into the hills. When they heard the news, his neighbors said, "Such bad luck, to lose your only horse." "Maybe," the farmer replied.

The next morning the horse returned, bringing with it three other wild horses. "How wonderful," the neighbors exclaimed. "Maybe," replied the old man.

The following day, the farmer's son tried to ride one of the wild horses, but he was thrown and broke his leg. The neighbors again came to offer their sympathy. "Maybe," answered the farmer.

The day after, soldiers came to the village to draft young men into the army. Seeing that the son's leg was broken, they passed him by. The neighbors congratulated the farmer on how well things had turned out. "Maybe," said the farmer.

And then, of course, the young village men were killed in the war and the farmer's son, even with a limp, was the only able-bodied young man remaining in the village. The farmer and his son prospered. When his neighbors praised his fortune, well, you know how the farmer replied. "Maybe."

From *How to Live Well with Chronic Pain and Illness*

by Toni Bernhard

Living at ease with life's uncertainty is difficult enough without the added challenge of chronic illness. Will we ever be able to do the things we treasured so much before we got sick? Will the people we meet treat us with understanding and compassion? What does the future hold? We just don't know.

Since uncertainty is an inevitable part of human experience, the quality of our lives will improve dramatically if we can find a way to make peace with it. When I awake each morning, I try to reflect on how I can't know what the day has in store for me, especially with regard to my health. Then I set the intention to greet it nonetheless with as much caring attention, compassion, and open-hearted curiosity as I can muster.

Did you have a moment this week of recognizing the open-ended possibilities in your life?

Give yourself a gold leaf!

Transformation

by Julianne Lepp

We recall our connection
In the seed sprouting
In the whisper of wind
In the new green wood

We inhabit a world of changes

We have not lost hope
In the dust of the desert
In the rush of the wave
In the rise of the mountain

We are part of it all

We remember the cycle
In the promise of blossoms
In the dying leaves
In the bare branches

We are becoming, we are letting go.

Don't Know Mind

by Zen Master Bon Soeng of the Kwan Um School of Korean Zen

This basic teaching we have is Don't-Know Mind. We want to know, we think we know, we think we're supposed to know. There's all of this bias toward knowing. But we don't really know. We have this radical teaching—how about admitting the truth that we don't know and go from there. If we really live that, it changes everything.

Don't-Know doesn't mean stupid. It means What Is It? Suddenly our eyes are open, we're vibrating with energy because we wonder, "What?" . . . rather than, "Oh yeah, I know that!"

Suzuki Roshi's quote was, "A beginner's mind is wide open and questioning. An expert's mind is closed." So this Not-Knowing actually gives us life. It gives vibrancy and energy to the world we live in. This kind of I-Know shuts everything down and we get stuck. Yet all the signals from everything around us say we're supposed to know. The competition is who knows the most but look at the result.

We fill our minds up with all this stuff, and it gets stale and dead. Not knowing is what opens us up and comes alive. In Buddhism and in Zen, there are a lot of different ways to talk about this very same thing. Sometimes we call it Don't-Know Mind, sometimes we call it Beginner's Mind, sometimes we call it Before Thinking Mind.

It all comes down to this, (Zen Master hits the floor). Clear it away. Return to zero. What do we see, what do we smell, what do we taste, what do we touch? Everything is truth. What we know blocks the truth. Returning to not knowing opens us up.

Journal Prompts
Dancing with Unpredictability

A chronic illness is not difficult to live with because it is endless. It is difficult to live with because it is unpredictable. But like grief, every flare ends, and though the looming threat is constant, you will learn to live beside it. A shadow of mixed blessings. It does not heal as wounds do, but it teaches you of your own strength till you wear it like a battle scar.

LANCALI, *I FELL IN LOVE WITH HOPE*

- Does the quote above ring true for you? In what ways? In what ways not?

- What have you learned about dancing with unpredictability in the time you have been ill? Do you feel that it has taught you your own strength?

Reflection Questions
Change and Unpredictability

Letting there be room for not knowing is the most important thing of all. When there's a big disappointment, we don't know if that's the end of the story. It may just be the beginning of a great adventure. Life is like that. We don't know anything. We call something bad; we call it good. But really we just don't know.

PEMA CHODRON

- What do you find most challenging about the changes and unpredictability of illness?

- How has your illness changed over time?

- What would you want to say to your friends and family to help them understand when you need to change plans for health reasons?

- How does the Buddhist teaching of Not Knowing resonate with you?

Playlist for Unpredictability

A Little Soon to Say by Jackson Browne

Uncertainty by Tow'rs

Unpredictable by Angelica Hale

Unpredictable by Celeste Buckingham

Everything Must Change by Nina Simone

Learning to Sit with Not Knowing by Carrie Newcomer

Hang On by Guster

Hey Stranger by Phish

Year-Long Winter by Johnny Flynn

11
Caregiving

To love a person is to see all of their magic, and to remind them of it when they have forgotten.

Anonymous

In the spring, the pollinators are buzzing around lush blossoms. Gardeners take time to water, nurture, and care for their plants. Caring relationships are similar: caregivers are invested in their patients or loved ones, and it takes time and intention to help them flourish.

Caregiving is challenging physically, mentally, and spiritually—it takes a toll to be in charge of another person's well-being. Unless you are already a professional caregiver, there can be a steep learning curve when finding yourself in this role. How do you care for yourself while learning how to care for another? What spiritual practices might you find to support you in this work?

Self-care isn't a luxury. When you are pouring out energy while caring for another, you need a way to recover and re-energize yourself. Self-care looks different for each person. If you're an extrovert, you might enjoy coffee with friends or a yoga or mindfulness class. If you're an introvert, you might enjoy a coffee date with yourself, going to the library, or a quiet walk. Self-care isn't selfish: burnout is a real danger in caregiving, and practicing self-compassion and self-care makes it that much easier to be available to the person you are helping.

Caregiving is especially hard when the caregiver is also living with chronic illness. It is difficult to care for your own health needs when you are driving to appointments, washing clothes, tracking medications, and everything else. The stress of caregiving can impact relationships between couples, family, and friends. It is important to have strong communication between the receiver and giver so both can express their needs. This isn't always easy when it is a loved one suffering, but good boundaries and communication ease potential resentments and stress on your relationship.

In this section, you are invited to explore spiritual resources to support your role as a caregiver. Just as caregivers give their time, they must also have a time to receive their own care and support. To care for others, you have to also care for yourself!

Every one of us needs to show how much we care for each other and, in the process, care for ourselves.

PRINCESS DIANA

Who Cares for the Caregiver?

Julianne's Story

> There are only four kinds of people in the world:
> Those who have been caregivers. Those who are
> currently caregivers. Those who will be caregivers,
> and those who will need a caregiver.
>
> ROSALYN CARTER

In a recent conversation with my older sister, I was reminded of the heavy load of caregiving that fell into her lap all at once in her early thirties. Being a caregiver can happen unexpectedly due to a sudden illness, injury, or other unexpected circumstances. This happened when my mother, who lived in the midlands of South Carolina, was diagnosed with lung cancer in 1999. I lived in Georgia and my brother lived in Florida, so we could only help so much from afar. My sister, Gregg, still lived in South Carolina and ended up taking the brunt of caretaking for both my mother and our grandmother Nana, who had been diagnosed with Alzheimer's.

Like many caregivers, Gregg already had a lot of stressors on her plate. She was a newly divorced mom with a young son, and she had recently started a new teaching job and struggled with handling her own chronic health conditions. Her unexplained ailments had begun in her teens. Over the years she was diagnosed with joint and connective tissue pain, irritable bowel syndrome, gastroesophageal reflux disease, Graves' disease, and hypothyroid disease. Once she became a caregiver, she would spend hours driving each week to check on and help care for my mother and Nana. Between full-time teaching and parenting, she wore herself out trying to also meet the needs of loved ones.

Both my mother and Nana were initially in denial of their illnesses. My mother was certain the cancer couldn't be as bad as the doctors predicted, and Nana was terrified of having Alzheimer's like her own grandmother. Nana's grandmother had literally been kept in the family attic due to her illness and the "embarrassment" it caused the family. Nana told horror stories of chasing her grandmother down the street when she was only wearing a slip. There were no care homes then, and many who suffered were locked away due to a lack of options and the sense of shame associated with dementia or Alzheimer's. Nana's own siblings were too ashamed to keep bringing her to church as her symptoms became more obvious. They were afraid that she might act out in some embarrassing way.

When Nana's condition deteriorated to the point that she got lost driving to an appointment that didn't exist and tried to give the newspaper delivery person a huge check, the family had to move her to assisted care. It was not an easy transition for her to lose her home and driving privileges: she was scared and confused much of the time. Nana would call Gregg every day, sometimes in the middle of the night, wondering when she could go home and who these people were who were taking care of her. At the same time, my mother's symptoms also worsened, and she would lean on Gregg about her fears of dying and the panic she felt from her reduced lung capacity and health. It was too much for one person. Who cares for the caregiver?

Gregg said she doesn't regret her years of caregiving, but she knew even then what a toll it took on her body, spirit, and emotions. When I asked her how she cared for herself, she laughed at first. There was little if any time for her to go to her own doctor's appointments or find time for self-care. She did find some time to grab moments for herself: she read books and would stay up late reading for pleasure. She would take a long soaking bath and listen to music. For caregivers, finding even small moments of peace can be a lifeline. These moments can be as simple as taking a moment in silence alone or ordering a favorite meal or treat to savor quietly. While she considered it an honor to care for her loved ones, in retrospect she sees that she needed to care for herself as well.

Having spiritual and emotional support along with physical help can also be key. I work full time as a minister and live in a multigenerational household, and I do my own share of caregiving at times. I try to find balance between my own care and those of my loved ones, but there are simply some weeks when my own needs get put to the side. Communities of support like congregations, support groups, or interest groups can give needed support to both the caregiver and receiver. Hiring help or finding additional aid from family and friends can also help avoid caregiver burnout and resentment.

As a Unitarian Universalist minister, I believe in the worthiness and dignity of each person. Both the caregiver and recipient deserve love and care. When I talk with caregivers, I always ask them one simple and fundamental question. Where are you finding support?

Spiritual Practice

For Caregivers

Taking care of yourself is probably the most important spiritual practice as a caregiver. As the popular phrase goes, put on your own oxygen mask first before caring for others. Caregiving can be stressful and draining if you aren't caring for yourself as well. Here are some thoughts for spiritual practices of renewal:

Movement

You may feel and sleep better if you find ways to move your body and exercise to a level that works for your body. Movement is not only good for physical health; it also benefits spiritual and mental health as well.

Mindful Eating

When you are busy with caregiving, it is hard to find time to slow down and enjoy your meals. Taking time away from your caregiving to eat alone or with plenty of time to savor the meal will help you connect with and enjoy your food.

Take "You" Time

For example, make time to read, do a puzzle, listen to music, paint, do crafts, or play games—even if you can only do it for a few minutes a day. If you like to go to activities, do certain hobbies, or take classes, find a way to take time to do that for yourself. Remind yourself that you have a life of your own to enjoy.

Joy and Play

Attending a play or concert that you'd enjoy will take you out of the everyday tasks of caretaking. Finding time to connect to playfulness, laughter, and lighter emotions is important. You can read more in the Play chapter in this book.

Caregiving can be rigorous. You are more than your role and you deserve to take these important breaks.

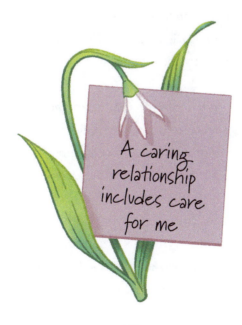

A caring relationship includes care for me

Caretaking and Making Space for Me

Selika's Story

I've been an academic for many years, but caretaking has defined me in so many ways. While I have chronic ailments like asthma and a heart murmur, chronic illness has affected me more in my role as a caretaker.

I'm a Black, cisgender woman in my fifties who grew up in a Black Catholic community in the 60s and 70s; there were very traditional roles expected of me as a woman and within my own family. In Southeastern Louisiana Creole culture, it was fine for my elder brother to play football, but as the eldest daughter I was expected to look after our home and my youngest brother Vincent. I did this from age seven to age thirty. Vincent had severe autism and a pervasive developmental disorder and needed looking after constantly. With this kind of responsibility, I didn't have sleepovers and activities like band trips that a normal childhood would entail. I couldn't do things after school because I needed to be home to take care of him.

One time he ran down the road naked and headed straight toward the sugar cane and strawberry fields near our home. By the time I caught up with him, most of the neighborhood was following to help out. Neighbors helped out neighbors when they could.

Caretaking was difficult. I never had any private space for myself: he'd burst into my room, so I had to change clothes in the bathroom. I used to have to keep the car keys under my pillow so Vincent wouldn't steal them. And when I went on dates, Vincent would sit in the back seat of the car. It affected who was willing to date me. It affected all aspects of my life. I took care of his hygiene and personal care, which became more challenging as he grew older. Eventually he was a tall man who weighed over 250 pounds, and he was much bigger than me. I learned to use tricks like promising him his favorite show or meal to help keep ahead of him. I really didn't get to live a life of my own until I was thirty.

I came out of that intensive caretaking with a sense of hypervigilance due to years of having to anticipate my brother's actions. I was always seen as "older" and more responsible than most people my age. The message I get now in my fifties is that I'm not a good daughter because my mother doesn't live with me. Though I share caretaking for my aging mother with family members, I've chosen for her not to live with me. I am also not willing to sacrifice my children to that role in the way I had to deal with growing up. And I'm learning now in my fifties to make space for myself. That might mean letting my children or husband walk the dog so I can have a quiet walk by myself. It means reading science fiction and paranormal books for fun and tending to my hydroponic garden. I've recently gotten an electric violin and have been reconnecting with music.

I have shifted my ideas about what caretaking looks like, and it looks like self-care.

Enough

by Julianne Lepp

Grief settles in my body like an unwanted guest,
clawing at joints, claiming all my attention.
I would shake it away like a wet dog if I could.

Gently grasping aching fingers,
the way I held your hand yesterday.
My hand cradles the other.
Remembering how my hand was cool
and yours quite warm.

Sitting at your bedside,
I watched your chest rise and fall in its uncertain way.
The time was closing and my offerings were small.
Simple songs, familiar words, and a comforting hand.

Touch and hearing are the last senses to go.

What is it that we have to offer one another?
We people who journey, laugh, and live
on this crowded ball of dirt called Earth?

We rush into this world with wailing wonder,
the journey ahead full of mystery and possibility.
Time narrows, decisions are made,
and yet moments like these are what stand apart.
Hands held at bedsides.

Humans are little animated balls of stardust,
hard to predict, prone to mistakes and messes.
We enter and leave the world on our own,
though not truly alone. Like trees in a forest,
our lives are intertwined with all of life.

One hand cradling another.
A breath. A song. A few words.
That is what we can offer one another.
And perhaps that is enough.

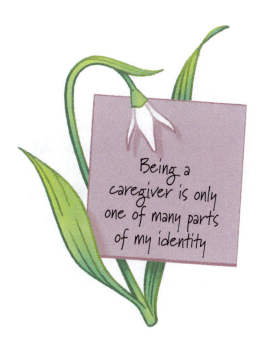

Being a caregiver is only one of many parts of my identity

Have you been taking moments to care for yourself, allowing yourself to acknowledge the gifts and challenges of this work? Even noticing is a step toward mindfulness!

Give yourself a gold leaf!

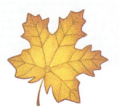

Too often we underestimate the power of a touch, a smile, a kind word, a listening ear, an honest compliment, or the smallest act of caring, all of which have the potential to turn a life around.

LEO BUSCAGLIA, *LIVING, LOVING AND LEARNING*

Prayer in Action

by Jane Ellen Mauldin in
Glory, Hallelujah! Now Please Pick Up Your Socks

A number of years ago, my brother lay dying in the hospital. He spent days in the intensive care unit while members of my family, including my mother, sat for many long hours on chairs in the hallway outside his room. Among visitors who came to share the vigil was a member of our church.

"How are you doing?" the friend asked.

My mother was too exhausted to tell anything but the truth. "I'm tired," she said. "I'm very, very tired. I'm too tired to even pray anymore."

"But don't you see," her friend replied, "your very presence here is a prayer."

There are times when all the words fail us, all forms seem hollow, and no one out there or inside seems to be listening. At those times, our presence, just our presence, is prayer. Our bodies, our actions, become our prayer, our connection to God, whatever God may be.

Journal Prompts
Caregiving

Whether you are caregiving part time or full time, it can be both rewarding and challenging. You are invited to gently explore all or a few of these prompts and follow where your thoughts take you.

- I define caregiving as . . .

- When I am overwhelmed, I show myself grace by . . .

- My favorite time of day with the one I care for is . . .

- Some of the thoughts I think over and over are . . .

- If I was my friend, I would tell myself . . .

After journaling, give yourself time to process. Sit quietly with what came up in your thoughts and emotions, and perhaps explore them further by writing more or by talking with a friend or support person.

From *Turning Suffering Inside Out*

by Darlene Cohen

When I was very ill and needed help with the simplest activities like washing my hair, I found it draining to be helped by people whom I constantly had to reassure that they were doing enough, doing things the right way, seeing me often enough. They paid much more attention to their ideas of "helping a person in need" than to me personally. How refreshing and soothing it was to be tended to by people who were able to approach me directly, without ideas about what they were doing with me, without using me to define who they were at that moment. This was not a subtle difference to me at the time; it was roaringly blatant. The two approaches produced a dramatically different impact on my energy level.

Caregiving often calls us to lean into love we didn't know possible.

TIA WALKER

Reflection Questions
Caregiving

My caregiver mantra is to remember: the only control you have is over the changes you choose to make.

NANCY L. KRISEMAN, *THE MINDFUL CAREGIVER*

- What self-care are you going to do for yourself today?

- What do you enjoy most about caregiving? What have been some of the hardest moments?

- What memories or history of caregiving do you have in your family and life, and how do you think they affect how you approach caregiving?

- Are there lessons or gifts that arise for you from caring for another person?

Playlist for Caregiving

Breathe by Faith Hill

One Voice by the Wailin' Jennys

I Will Carry You by Ellie Holcomb

Ain't No Mountain High Enough by Marvin Gaye and
Tammi Terrell

Hold my Hand by Hootie & the Blowfish

Soon You'll Get Better by Taylor Swift

I'll Get By by Avi Kaplan

Good Job by Alicia Keys

12

Shame and Being Enough

May the light be upon me,
May I feel in my bones that I'm enough.

Pink, "I Am Here"

Spring is a season of new life and overflowing beauty in the natural world, and yet, paradoxically, it can be a time when those of us facing physical challenges can feel that we are out of step with the season, and even out of step with the world. We may not feel the springing up of new life in our bones; when friends are rushing outside to enjoy the milder weather, we may still be huddled in blankets on the couch. These experiences are fertile ground for feelings of shame and inadequacy.

Because our culture does not honor those who are disabled or differently abled and celebrates health and youth, we may feel judged by others, and by ourselves, as not enough: not enough energy, not enough strength, not enough capacity. One way to think about shame is that it is an attack by the part of us that has internalized what we *think* the judgements of others are, which we then heap on ourselves. Shame is an extremely painful emotion, even dangerous, since it can lead to depression and self-hatred.

In working with internalized judgments, the first step is recognizing the attack, since self-judgment often happens unconsciously. The second step is to intentionally cultivate kindness toward ourselves, both for the challenges we face and for the pain of the self-judgement itself.

Whatever our condition, whatever our ability, we are enough. Coming to know that, deeply, is one of the greatest challenges and spiritual practices of chronic illness.

Experiencing shame can itself feel shameful, so it's easy to bury the reality of how shame is influencing us. But bringing it out in the open and realizing how much of it is culturally conditioned can lead to freedom and even joy, regardless of our physical challenges. Now that is the energy of spring!

This chapter explores the tender territory of shame and offers support for the journey toward a life where we are not as powerfully subject to shame's stories about ourselves.

> Many people feel that it's somehow their fault when they become chronically ill. They see it as a personal failing on their part. We live in a culture that reinforces this view by bombarding us with messages about how, if we'd just eat this food or engage in that exercise, we need never worry about our health... The first few years after I got sick, I was "chronically embarrassed" about not being able to recover my health.
>
> TONI BERNHARD, *HOW TO LIVE WELL WITH CHRONIC PAIN AND ILLNESS*

Shame, or the School Nurse
Who Lives on Inside Me

Florence's Story

It is late spring, and every morning I see children walking by under the big old trees that overhang the sidewalks, on the way to their last days of school before a summer of freedom. I see them and remember what it was like to be headed to school as a child, groggy and rushed. In my memory, I am nearly always running late.

My feelings about school were mixed: on the one hand, I loved learning and reading. But on the other hand, it was hard to get up so early and be in a classroom all day, and there were the inevitable interpersonal stresses: the shifting alliances, the class bullies, and the ways I often felt different, strange, or left out. Some days these stresses would spill over into nausea, dizziness, or other somatic responses, or I would be sick with some virus, and I would be sent to see the school nurse, in her small, quiet, dark room with a single bed.

What I remember from those visits was a pervasive sense that she (it was always a woman) would think I was faking illness, no matter how terrible I felt. I desperately wanted to be running a fever so she would believe me. I don't know where this feeling came from, except that perhaps I longed for a break from the classroom, to lie in that cool, quiet room for a while, and I was afraid that the nurse would sense my desire and send me back into the world.

It was much the same with my mother, when I felt too sick in the morning for my walk to school. I would think, "Will she believe me? Will she think I'm pretending to be sick?" And maybe I was, some days.

Now, decades later as an adult, I have a number of diagnosed conditions that limit what I can do, and which leave me often feeling quite legitimately terrible. But I still have the sense that someone is going to look over my shoulder, click their tongue disapprovingly, and tell me to just get up and stop faking it. Before my diagnosis this feeling was even stronger, because without a name for what I was experiencing, I was quite sure others would judge me—and sometimes they did. This is one of the unsung miseries of being sick with something that doesn't have a name. Only when I had a name for my condition did I have the courage to make needed changes in my life.

Doctors, insurance companies, and anyone with power over me will still trigger this inner story. In my work with others who are living with the challenges of chronic illness or disability, I often hear the same fear and shame. Toni Bernhard, in her book *How to Live Well with Chronic Pain and Illness*, describes this same feeling: "I was particularly concerned that they would think I was a malingerer—someone who feigns illness in order avoid work and other responsibilities."

There are names for that internalized authority figure that looks over our shoulders and tells us that we are faking it, we are weak, or we are failing. Sometimes it is called the Inner Critic or the Inner Judge. The Inner Judge comes from authority figures in childhood—a parent, an older sibling, teachers—or apparently, in my case, a school nurse. It is scathing in its judgment, even cruel.

It is well documented that age, gender, sexual orientation, weight, and race, among other identities, can make it more or less likely that we will experience undeserved judgments from medical providers, bosses, and others. If our symptoms are dismissed or downplayed by those with medical power over us, it can be life-threatening. (For example, my stepmother died because of a doctor's dismissal of her undiagnosed cancer symptoms, telling her that her extreme fatigue was because of her age.) These judgments from others can easily compound our own judgments of ourselves.

If you suddenly feel small and worthless, chances are you have just experienced an attack from the Inner Judge. If you find yourself thinking something that starts with "Everyone thinks I am . . ." or "Why are you . . ." you are probably experiencing an attack from the Inner Judge. Those of us with illness and pain can be judged by the culture and by others, so it's no wonder we judge ourselves as well.

In my years of consciously working with this part of myself and helping others with their own, what I have learned is that the first and most powerful step in no longer believing what the Inner Judge says is to name it when it is happening. Awareness itself is freeing. The words of the Inner Judge are not the truth of my situation, however convincing they may sound.

The spiritual teacher Byron Katie has two questions you can ask yourself when a judging or limiting thought is going through your head, and you can only answer yes or no to them. The first is, "Am I sure this is true?" If you say "yes" to that question (for example, "Yes, I am sure this illness is an excuse for not working as hard as others do"), then the second question is, "Am I absolutely sure this is true?" Sometimes you might even say yes to the second question, but nine times out of ten, you cannot be absolutely sure, especially since so many of the Inner Judge's opinions are ridiculous.

When I catch that I am judging myself, I can remember: I am no longer the child walking to school with all the confusions and vulnerabilities of childhood. I am no longer the child in that quiet nurse's office, hoping I can stay there just a little longer. I am an adult, doing the best I can with the circumstances of my life. Those circumstances include a rather dizzying array of health challenges. When I see my life that way, there is no room for disapproval. Only compassion, both for that child I was and for the person I am today.

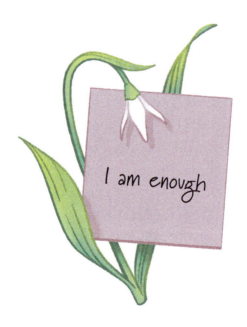

We Are Whole

by Beth Lefever in *Becoming: A Spiritual
Guide for Navigating Adulthood*

We are whole,
even in the broken places,
even where it hurts.

We are whole,
even in the broken places,
the places where fear impedes our full engagement with life;
where self-doubt corrupts our self-love;
where shame makes our faces hot and our souls cold.

We are whole,
even in those places where perfectionism blunts the joy
of full immersion into person, place, activity;
where "good enough" does not reside except in our silent
longings;
where our gaps must be fast-filled
with substance, accomplishment, or frenzied activity
lest they gape open and disgust.

We are whole
where we would doubt our own goodness, richness, fullness
and depth,
where we would doubt our own significance, our own
profoundness.

We are whole,

even in our fragility;
even where we feel fragmented, alone, insubstantial,
insufficient.

We are whole,
even as we are in process,
even as we stumble,
even as we pick ourselves up again,
for we are whole.

We are whole.

An affirmation

I am the expert on my own pain. I know that my experiences are real,
whether or not authority figures acknowledge it. I deserve to get the
rest and care I need, and I do not need to feel ashamed about it.

Spiritual Practice

A "Being Kind to Yourself" Retreat

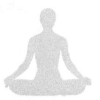

Kindness is a quality of mind we can cultivate toward ourselves as well as others. Many of us struggle to treat ourselves kindly. Having been conditioned throughout our lives to hold ourselves to impossible standards, we've become our own harshest critics. If you're quick to direct negative judgment at yourself, pause for a moment and imagine how it would feel if you spent the entire day being friendly, caring, and considerate to yourself.

TONI BERNHARD, *HOW TO LIVE WELL WITH CHRONIC PAIN AND ILLNESS*

Intentionally set aside a day or a part of a day to try this practice. Begin by asking yourself these questions: How would you treat a dear friend during this day, or a beloved and honored family member? What nice things would you do for them? How would you talk with them? How would you be kind?

Make a plan for how you will treat yourself. What would make you happiest? What would give you a sense of being cared for and nurtured?

Then explore what happens during the day, or part of the day, you set aside. You may encounter some resistance or self-judgment, but just keep exploring what it feels like to treat yourself well, even self-indulgently! You deserve it.

> What you do for yourself, any gesture of kindness, any gesture of gentleness, any gesture of honesty and clear seeing toward yourself, will affect how you experience your world. In fact, it will transform how you experience the world. What you do for yourself, you're doing for others, and what you do for others, you're doing for yourself.
>
> PEMA CHODRON, *COMFORTABLE WITH UNCERTAINTY*

Can you see yourself as a tree, in all your beautiful imperfection?

Give yourself a gold leaf!

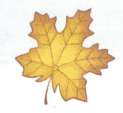

From *Sitting Pretty: The View from My Ordinary Resilient Disabled Body*

by Rebekah Taussig

When I was small and just learning how to do life in my body, I didn't hesitate, didn't hold back, didn't worry how it would look, didn't look for cues or ask for a line. . . . I was entirely free to *be*, driven by the innovation my body inspired. This is the wild emancipation I wish for all of us—a world where we are all free to be, to move, to exist in our bodies without shame; a world that isn't interested in making all of its humans operate in the exact same way; a world that instead strives to invite more, include more, imagine more. That world sees the humans existing on the margins and says, *You have what we want! What barriers can we remove so we can have you around? What do you need? How can we make that happen?*

The Healing Moment

by Elizabeth Tarbox in *Life Tides*

Each day I am newly reminded of my unworthiness: a dozen thoughts misspoken; another day when the good I do falls so far short of the good I could do; myriad small interchanges, moments of sharing that strain to the breaking point my desire to be generous, helpful, and kind; months of careful work lost by a moment's impatience, a careless word.

But when I am here at the edge of creation, breaking with the small tide over the sand, the need to do good rolls away; the question of what is right diminishes to insignificance and is easily borne away by the tiny waves. Here, where no words are spoken, none are misspoken.

I am with the broken stubble of the marsh grass that holds on through the wrecking wind and the burning flood. I am with the grains that mold themselves around everything, accepting even so unworthy a foot as mine, holding and shaping it until it feels that it belongs. I stand somewhere between truth and vision, and what I don't know ceases to embarrass me, because what I do know is that the water feels gentle like a lover's touch, and the sand welcomes it.

What I have done or failed to do has left no noticeable mark on creation. What I do or don't do is of no moment now. Now I am here and grateful to be touched, calmed, and healed by the immense pattern of the universe. And when I die, it will be an honor for my blood to return to the sea and my bones to become the sand. Reassured, I am called back to my life, to another day.

From "Ram Dass on Self-Judgment"

When you go out into the woods, and you look at trees, you see all these different trees. And some of them are bent, and some of them are straight, and some of them are evergreens, and some of them are whatever. And you look at the tree and you allow it. You appreciate it. You see why it is the way it is. You sort of understand that it didn't get enough light, and so it turned that way. And you don't get all emotional about it. You just allow it. You appreciate the tree.

The minute you get near humans, you lose all that. And you are constantly saying, "You're too *this*, or I'm too *this*." That judging mind comes in. And so I practice turning people into trees. Which means appreciating them just the way they are.

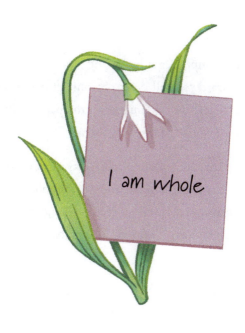

I am whole

Journal Prompts

Finding Freedom from Self-Judgment

Inspired by the work of Byron Katie

> You are taught that there is something wrong with you and that you're imperfect. But there isn't and you're not.
>
> CHERI HUBER

For this journal prompt, begin by jotting down some of the judgements you feel toward yourself due to chronic illness or pain. Just let your pen flow and get your judgments on the paper, without, if you can help it, judging yourself for having them.

Then choose one that feels particularly sticky or persuasive, write it again at the top of a page, and ask yourself the following questions, writing down the answers. This is an exercise designed to help loosen the hold the judgment has on your mind and heart.

- Is this true? (Write only "yes" or "no" rather than "no, but . . ." or "maybe.")

- Is it *absolutely* true? (Write only "yes" or "no" rather than "no, but . . ." or "maybe.")

- What would be the opposite of this judgement?

- What are three pieces of evidence from your own experience that there is some truth to the opposite of your judgement?

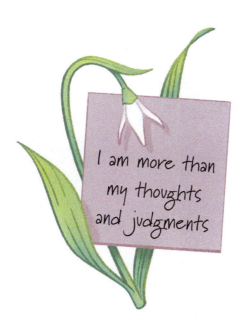

I am more than my thoughts and judgments

Reflection Questions

Shame and Being Enough

- What did your family and culture teach you about how you "should" be?

- Does chronic illness, pain, or disability mean that you can't live up to those societal standards? How so?

- Have you experienced judgments from others—family, friends, doctors—around your condition? Tell one story.

- What have you found most helpful when you notice that you are judging yourself?

- What does it feel like when you know you're enough?

Playlist for Being Enough

Just as You Are by Lea Morris

Flaws and All by Beyoncé

This Is Me by Benj Pasek and Justin Paul, sung by the cast of *The Greatest Showman*

Who Says by Selena Gomez & the Scene

Who You Are by Jessie J

How Could Anyone by Libby Roderick

Enough by Sara Bareilles

I Know This Rose Will Open by Mary Grigolia, sung by Ann Hamilton

My Hands Are Strong Enough by Lea Morris

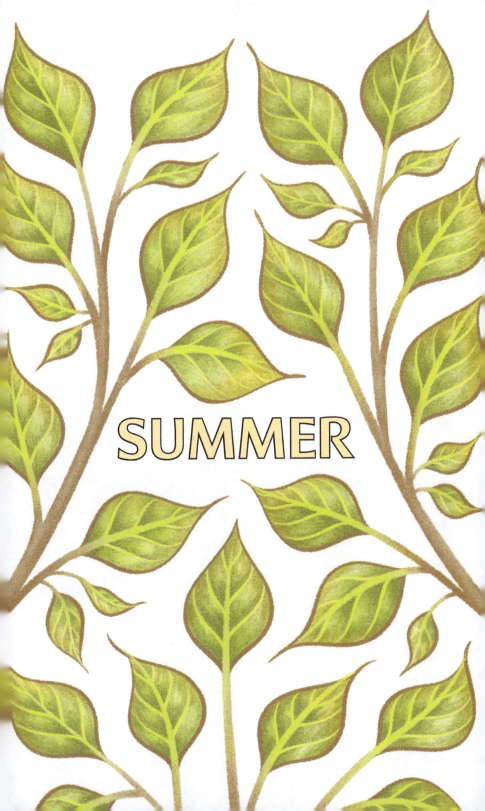

SUMMER

SUMMER

By Julianne Lepp

Summer is a time when I spend a lot of time reflecting and slowing down to examine my life. As Allison Alexander writes in *Super Sick: Making Peace with Chronic Illness,* "Those of us with chronic pain have something unique to offer, not in spite of our pain, but because of it."

When I was diagnosed with rheumatoid arthritis, I was hurting and scared, so I reached out to others online for support. It seemed like my whole world had narrowed and the future looked bleak. What kind of future was I going to have, and how would I make it through the challenges ahead? Luckily, I met my co-writer and fellow Unitarian Universalist minister, Florence, through an online forum for health concerns. Her friendship, support, and shared work on this project have been an unexpected gift. It has been a chance to explore the spiritual dimensions of living with chronic illness and pain in a focused way.

During our interviews and work on this book, I have felt so inspired by people's stories. Every day, people who live with chronic illness are incredibly adaptive, creative, determined, and strong. Living in adversity creates different kinds of gifts. Just to get up out of bed in the morning might be an Olympic accomplishment for someone. Doing the dishes or showing up for work on time can feel worthy of a

Summer has many lessons for taking care of beleaguered bodies that need support, rest and joy. What are the gifts of the season of summer that you long for?

In this section you will find reflections on the themes of summer: beauty and bliss, rest and sabbath, play and laughter, isolation and connection. May these resources support you in transformation and joy and remind you to rest and connect deeply with nature, yourself, and others. And mostly, may you know that you're not alone on this journey.

Ah, summer! The season when worry steps aside, delight takes over, and every day is as good as the amount of time spent outdoors. It's a chance to swim past the breakers, take outdoor showers, hold court from a pool float, or rely on nothing but your wits, a pineapple, rum, and a blender to make the most of an afternoon. When the only imperative is to unwind, unplug, and open up to a day of possibilities, you know you're going to have fun.

MARNIE HANEL, *SUMMER: A COOKBOOK*

13
Rest and Sabbath

The etymological root of the word Sabbath means to stop—doing, producing, thinking, to stop time, in essence, to allow oneself the void in which to receive, instead of constantly striving "to be."

Savannah Blaze Lee, *The Gospel of Mary*

Summer is known as a time to slow down and rest. There are iconic pictures of people dozing in hammocks or relaxing on the beach. While rest is something most people value, our society struggles with prioritizing time for rest and sleep. According to the National Sleep Foundation, up to 30% of adults in the US struggle with insomnia, and a similar percentage report sleeping an average of less than seven hours a night. We work hard and play hard, and our health pays the price.

Getting enough sleep is key to better health, and getting good rest is also important for our mental and spiritual health. Finding that balance in a busy world can be tricky. One of the most powerful ways to honor your need for rest is to have good boundaries around your energy and time. You have the right to say no to tasks, requests, and demands that aren't in your best interest. Say yes to what you do need, and feel empowered to say no to what does not serve you.

Sabbath is an intentional, recurring time set aside for rest. It is a time to view rest as spiritual practice and through a spiritual lens. For people prone to pushing themselves past their limits—a common impulse for those with chronic health issues—turning rest into a mindful recurring practice can help it feel more rewarding and relaxing. Rather than waiting until your body forces a halt and then feeling frustrated or guilty about it, make rest a part of your routine that you can sink into and enjoy.

In her book *Rest Is Resistance: A Manifesto,* Tricia Hersey argues that overworking can be toxic. In a culture that is hyper-focused on output, Hersey lifts up the value of inner calm and better health that can come with enough rest and sabbath time. It is good to prioritize your energy and health so that you can lead a balanced life.

This chapter invites you to embrace the power of rest and listen deeply to the needs of your body. When is the last time you felt rested? What practices might support more sabbath and rest in your life?

It's precisely those who are busiest who most need to give themselves a break.

Pico Iyer, *The Art of Stillness*

Rest in a "Type A" World

Julianne's Story

In my life, I have often considered "I am Superman" by R.E.M. to be my theme song. The refrain *I am Superman and I can do anything* was important to my identity of being completely self-sufficient. While this wasn't the healthiest notion, it was one I cleaved to for many years. I felt affirmed by being capable, productive, and energetic. No matter what happened, I thought, I was strong enough to take it.

It was quite the wakeup call when I discovered that chronic illness doesn't let you power through everything and that high performance and long days have a cost. Rest is essential, as is work and life balance. If I don't make time for rest, my body will make me take it by getting sick or having a flare.

During the early onset of my illness, I found that on my day off I'd have to spend the whole day on the couch resting. My rheumatoid arthritis was flaring and my pain levels were out of control, making fatigue and brain fog hard to manage. My day off became my recovery day from work, and also a day for my body to adjust to the nausea and fatigue from the strong medications I had to take. Thankfully, I have had some improvements over time. I adjusted my medicine and my diet and tried to manage my stress. These changes helped my quality of life significantly, which also helped my energy levels.

The reality of chronic illness is that for the rest of my life, I will need to make space for rest. There will be times when I need to try different medications or therapy, times when I can rely on my body and times when I can't. Some days I feel perfectly normal and full of energy, but most days I have to watch myself. Activities that used to be easy will tire my body out or cause soreness or a flare. Stress is a trigger for pain and flares, which then lead to a need for more rest. Yet most of my illness is not visible to others. So I have to be the one to protect my own rest time and my own need for recovery.

We live in a type A world, where being productive and busy is the gold standard. The first question people often ask is, "What do you do?" Whereas there aren't many gold stars being handed out for taking a midday nap or deciding to take sabbath time.

One of the most healing spaces that I have found is right in my front yard labyrinth and native garden. Putting down my phone and being present in a moment of rest feels like such a gift. Quietly sitting on my patio with my feet up and head back, I can watch the sway of coneflowers in the wind and hear the soft buzz of bees and other pollinators in the garden. There is a goldfinch that loves to grasp the head of my tall sunflowers, digging out seeds with its beak. A pair of monarchs flits across my labyrinth seeking out the hyssop in bloom. My breath slows and my mind stops racing.

Even five minutes away from my to-do list or the needs of others lets me prioritize the rest my body needs. Tricia Hersey writes in *Rest Is Resistance*, "Release the shame you feel when resting. It does not belong to you." I don't have to be Superman; I just need to be super at listening to my body. I need to recognize the value of myself and the value of rest.

I still need more healthy rest in order to work at my best. My health is the main capital I have and I want to administer it intelligently.

ERNEST HEMINGWAY

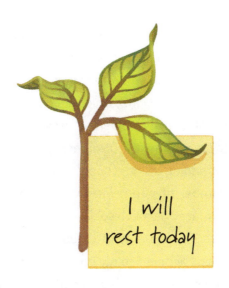

Rest and Play Are What I Need

Ehren's Story

I am a white, cisgender, queer male with allergies to dairy and gluten. Currently, I'm a senior in high school and will soon be eighteen years old. I'm an introvert and live with autism, anxiety, and depression. I find that I need a lot of rest and time away from social situations so that I don't get overwhelmed.

Like a lot of teenagers, I spend a lot of time in my room playing video games or on tech. I have accommodations at school so that I can take my tests in quieter spaces, and I eat my lunch in a quiet space near my counselor instead of in the loud and chaotic lunchroom. I have to be careful with certain foods due to sensory issues. I have IBS and also GERD, which affects my diet. I miss a lot of school now that I'm taking in-person classes. Everything is also compounded by general anxiety disorder and some sedentariness from years of attending online school.

I have a number of peers with worse conditions, and I'm grateful I haven't faced as much social stigma as I've seen others deal with. But there are plenty of embarrassing situations, like when I have gas or people find my bowel issues gross. It can be awkward, and there are some academic and social disadvantages to missing so much school. I also spend a lot of time on my own, since I can't deal with the noise of crowds or overlapping noises. I try to manage my IBS and GERD with a careful diet, with consideration for stomach issues and allergies. I do regular physical therapy and chiropractic care, and I eat simply, mainly vegetables, meat, and rice. I do this because of my sensitivity

From *Rest Is Resistance: A Manifesto*

by Tricia Hersey

You were not just born to center your entire existence on work and labor. You were born to heal, to grow, to be of service to yourself and community, to practice, to experiment, to create, to have space, to dream, and to connect. . . .

I want us to understand that nuance is freeing and freedom. There is no such thing as cookie-cutter healing. Everyone brings with them an origin story, a history, and identities that are interconnected. There is room to rest in the freedom of managing your own deprogramming journey. It is never either/or and always both/and. You don't have to grind, hustle, accept burnout as normal, and be in a constant state of exhaustion and sleep deprivation. You don't have to kill yourself spiritually or physically to live a fruitful life. This connection work is about restoring, remembering, reimagining, reclaiming, reparations, and redemption. Learning to make a way out of no way and seeing to the other side of trauma. It is believing you are worthy of rest because you are alive. Our bodies and souls want to be well, to heal, to be rested, and to be free from the hold productivity has over our lives. We are worthy now of rest, care, and space. We are worthy now of living in a place that respects our bodies for what they are: a divine dwelling.

Journal Prompts
Sacred Rest

In Saundra Dalton-Smith's book *Sacred Rest: Recover Your Life, Renew Your Energy, Restore Your Sanity,* she writes, "The body tells its story in stillness. When we are physically active, we focus on the motion without sensing the conversation going on inside of us. In stillness, we can recognize when movement is no longer serving us well."

- What story does your body tell in stillness?

- What happens when you slow down and listen to your body?

- What would it be like to listen to your body more often?

- When do you practice stillness and rest?

I loafe and invite my soul,
I lean and loafe at my ease observing a spear of summer grass . . .

WALT WHITMAN, *LEAVES OF GRASS*

What Is My New Normal?

by Angel L. McKenzie in . . . *surprise I have a chronic illness* . . .

Throughout most of my MS journey, I was intent on not changing a thing about my life, but instead maintaining my already established status quo. As I grew older and just a smidgen wiser, I learned that things change and change is okay; it can signify growth. My status quo was no longer going to work in my life, and I needed to establish a new "normal."

My new normal involved me understanding that I am superwoman (heck yeah, I am superwoman), but even superwoman needs to rest. I have learned that my worth should not be tied to my inability to do something as a result of my MS. I will admit that the last statement is the hardest thing for me to truly believe, but I will still continue to speak it and claim it for myself. I work a regular 40-hour work week but ensure to place sporadic days off in my schedule to recoup, or even call in when my body tells me I need to. I attend my kids' events and ensure to keep myself cool when those events involve the 3-digit Texas heat (the Texas heat can be so utterly disrespectful sometimes). I nurture my marriage and ensure to communicate with my husband when I am not feeling well. I understand that my mood swings and introverted personality cause me to expend an exorbitant amount of energy when engaging people. Knowing this, I work to not fill my days with an absurd number of events that require my full attention (at least when I can control my schedule).

From *Loving Our Own Bones: Disability Wisdom and the Spiritual Subversiveness of Knowing Ourselves Whole*

by Julia Watts Belser

Jewish tradition describes Shabbat as a foretaste of the world to come, a little touch of paradise, a promise. But I am not content to wait. I'm not content to put off gentleness and generosity. I'm not content to leave intact a world whose pace pushes certain bodies and minds to the margins, a world that runs roughshod over anyone who can't perform to a high-pitched standard. That's part of what I keep, when I keep Shabbos—a commitment to building and dreaming a different way of being. For those few hours, I feel it in my bones. I taste its sweetness on my tongue. A world that offers each of us enough, that gives us all the space to savor. A world that values us for who we are, not just for all that we have done. A world that teaches us to sink into the slow, to linger over twilight, to tune our hearts to a different kind of time.

The Map You Make Yourself

by Jan Richardson in *Circle of Grace*

You have looked
at so many doors
with longing,
wondering if your life
lay on the other side.

For today,
choose the door
that opens
to the inside.

Travel the most ancient way
of all:
the path that leads you
to the center
of your life.

No map
but the one
you make yourself.

No provision
but what you already carry
and the grace that comes

TEND TO YOUR SPIRIT

to those who walk
the pilgrim's way.

Speak this blessing
as you set out
and watch how
your rhythm slows,
the cadence of the road
drawing you into the pace
that is your own.

Eat when hungry.
Rest when tired.
Listen to your dreaming.
Welcome detours
as doors deeper in.

Pray for protection.
Ask for guidance.
Offer gladness
for the gifts that come,
and then
let them go.

Do not expect
to return
by the same road.
Home is always
by another way,
and you will know it

not by the light
that waits for you

but by the star
that blazes inside you,
telling you
where you are
is holy
and you are welcome
here.

*Are you giving yourself time to recover and rest
without shame? Are you listening to the needs of
your body? Even a small nap in the car counts.*

Give yourself a gold leaf!

Reflection Questions

Rest and Sabbath

- What time of day would you benefit from a short pause or rest, if possible?

- Is rest elusive or obtainable? Do you feel comfortable giving yourself time to rest?

- What are the messages about resting and honoring your body that you find helpful? What are some messages that you might let go?

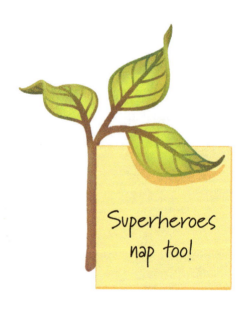

Playlist for Rest and Sabbath

Daydream by Wallace Collection

Lullaby by Tasha

I'm Tired by Labrinth and Zendaya

Only Time by Enya

Rest Life by Tricia Hersey

Rest by Michael Kiwanuka

Sitting on the Dock of the Bay by Otis Redding

Wild Mountain Thyme by Celtic Woman

Sleep by Blackalicious

A Chance to Rest by Lena Raine

Leisure Gardening by Lullatone

Down by the Water by The Drums

14

Beauty and Bliss

Remember there is always something

besides our own misery.

Linda Hogan

Summer is a lovely time. There is a luxuriant, sensuous quality to this season: warmth that allows for walking barefoot, the joy of a sunny morning, maybe even an echo of the ease of childhood.

Nonetheless, when the body is hurting, the beauty of summer (or any season) can feel infinitely far away. Other people are hiking among the flowers in the mountains, while some of us are confined inside or can only dimly imagine travel. Or we might be limited by our finances or caretaking responsibilities. It's hard not to feel resentful or envious of those well enough to go out and experience magnificent places. How can we find beauty in the middle of our difficult lives?

Most people tend to think that beauty is outside us, something that falls on our eyes or ears like a benediction. But what if finding beauty is instead a spiritual practice, one that can be cultivated the way one waters a pot of flowers on a front porch? What if we cultivated beauty with the same commitment as anything else we do for our physical and emotional well-being?

The Zen teacher Darlene Cohen taught a class for those with chronic pain called Suffering and Delight. She emphasized that finding delight—a close cousin of beauty—can be an antidote to pain. More recent research has shown that savoring experiences—stopping and really taking in beauty or pleasure—has many positive effects on the nervous system and the brain.

One of the secrets to finding beauty or bliss is, paradoxically, to understand how impermanent everything is, including ourselves. People who know they are dying sometimes find that they are overwhelmed by the simple bliss of being alive. They can't believe the rest of us can't see it, or that they missed it themselves for so long. In the John Ford movie *A Single Man*, the protagonist sees everything as if for the last time: the red lips of his secretary, the lovely face of a young man, the ocean waves, even a billboard. Walt Whitman, in his poem "Leaves of Grass," wrote: "Why, who makes much of a miracle? As to me I know of nothing else but miracles."

Beauty, awe, wonder, delight, bliss, ecstasy—these are all facets of the same jewel. In this chapter we celebrate this part of our humanity in its many forms, which can be a great gift in the long, hard seasons of living with a chronic condition. May beauty and bliss bless you, whatever your life may be.

People who truly know how to wonder don't expend a great deal of energy talking about it; they are off catching snowflakes on hot tongues. They're folding themselves in half to smell the sweet potatoes in the oven just one more time... I think awe is an exercise, both a doing and a being. It is a spiritual muscle of our humanity that we can only keep from atrophying if we exercise it habitually.

COLE ARTHUR RILEY, *THIS HERE FLESH*

Beauty in the Shadows

Florence's Story

Glory be to God for dappled things.

GERARD MANLEY HOPKINS

One summer I spent months in a serious bout of illness, mostly confined to my house. Finally I began to recover enough to venture out for slow walks, but because my life had narrowed down to the most basic tasks, I had stopped wearing glasses or contacts most of the time, and so my walks were both slow and blurry. And then something magical began to happen.

I live in an old neighborhood in a town renowned for its trees, a veritable urban forest. Every street is lined with huge old shade trees. In the years I have lived here, I have seen the trees in every permutation—bare limbs against a gray sky in winter, the first tentative blush of green in the early spring, the lush and nearly tropical summer, and for one or two glorious weeks, the hallucinatory colors of fall. But I had never, until that summer of illness, slowness, and blurred vision, really noticed the shadows.

I began to notice that on every sidewalk, on every street, whether in sunlight or at night under the streetlights, there was a constant play of shadow and light through the leaves. Once I began to see it, it was intoxicating, impossible not to see every time I went for a walk. In some places the shadow was solid, but mostly there was a dance of infinitely varied dapples, moving in the slightest breeze. I asked myself how I could have missed this wonder, which surely had been nearly everywhere I have walked in my life. It was at once so ordinary and so beautiful that it made me, at times, want to fall on my knees in awe and joy.

Would I have ever seen this without illness, without my sight being changed and blurred? I think not. And I laugh, realizing that loss and disability does indeed have its shadow side. I have been shown a glory that had been invisible to me, a living, changing, miraculous dance between such simple things—trees and leaves, light and surfaces, dappled shadows and my own eyes.

My mother was a person with an intense relationship with beauty and bliss. In the last year of her life, when she was 95 years old, I spent a lot of time with her. She had lost so much, things most of us desperately fear to lose: many of her memories, her life as a professor and researcher, her independence, her beautiful paintings, the bicycle she had ridden all over the world, her ability to read, to travel, or even to walk . . . The list of losses was very long, along with the many other indignities and losses of late old age.

And yet, every day I was with her I saw her overcome with joy from something. My hand in hers, an operatic aria on the radio, a tree blazing with red leaves against a deep blue sky, or even just rolling in her wheelchair across the threshold of the memory care where she lived, her house out into the big world she still loved so much.

I was amazed by her—by her inner and outer beauty, by her resilience, by her capacity for love and appreciation. By her willingness to say "yes" to her life even as it was so far from what she would wish for. I knew that she was severely compromised by dementia, but who she was, her qualities of heart, shone through so brightly, like the sun through dappled leaves.

"Shadow" is sometimes used pejoratively, but my mother showed me that even a shadowed life can be a beautiful life. And the trees in my neighborhood showed me that there is hidden beauty everywhere, even in the shadows on a cracked sidewalk, even—and maybe especially—in a season of illness.

Have you noticed one beautiful thing today?

Give yourself a gold leaf!

Broken Shellsong

by Julián Jamaica Soto in *Spilling the Light*

When I was a child, someone told me that
if you hold a seashell to your ear, you can hear
the ocean. When I was in middle school, I learned
that what you hear is not the ocean. It's just
the blood rushing through your ears. And that's fine.
But I still wonder if a broken seashell has any
good kind of song. The song of half a wave might
be a measure of grief. The Bay of Fundy when it
is empty. The bacteria flats in Yellowstone, steaming
copper and blue, smelling of sulfur and somehow
a cradle for life. Anklets of kelp forest. Even
mostly empty, the ocean cannot help but brim
with tokens of aliveness, reminders of beauty, and
the plain, unabashed assurance that broken things—
seashells, people, and times of love—have beauty all
their own, if we can dance in the offbeat, if we can
stand a little grit with the gorgeous gifts of
this wide world.

Good Lord, Thank You

Dawn's Story

I am an African American woman in my seventies, a daughter, mom, pastor, community organizer, and urban farmer. I have a servant spirit: my first inclination is to help.

As a teen I was diagnosed with a heart condition and seizure disorder, and I spent nearly a year in and out of the hospital. When I asked one of the doctors, "Is this going to kill me?" he told me that he didn't know. "You could die tomorrow or live to be one hundred." I was fifteen.

I made a bucket list shortly afterward. I didn't want to miss out on things if I died young; I wanted to live knowing I might die tomorrow. I didn't want to have a short life of foolish mistakes. Instead I have had a long life of well-thought-out mistakes!

When I was sick as a young person, my mother said I needed to think about someone besides myself. Sometimes challenges serve to show us who we are, show us what's important. When I was in the children's hospital, I saw other children with terrible burns and illnesses, worse than mine, and I realized that asking myself "What can I do?" made more sense than feeling sorry for myself and complaining.

As an adult I have also had psoriatic arthritis and diabetes. I have been able to use diet and lots of vegetables to control my blood sugar. The biggest part for me is not focusing on the pain and what I *can't* do, but what I *can* do. I'm slowing down now, in my seventies, but I'm still getting stuff done.

I had no intention of becoming an urban farmer, but I was teaching an after-school program in a building with no windows, and the kids thought peas came from the basement of the grocery store. We got a spot in a community garden and kiddie buckets and shovels from the Dollar Tree. I started learning to grow food, first from books, then from a master gardener program, then from the seniors in the community, and eventually from classes at the university.

Now I am the lead steward and "chief cook and bottle washer" of the Randolph Street Community Garden, where we teach people from the neighborhood, kids to seniors, how to grow their own food. We are such a ragtag group of folks. At one point a group of homeless men had a bed; they were homeless but not hungry. Seven languages are spoken in the garden.

The garden is such a peaceful place. I go to get centered there. When the news is crazy, I can sit in the garden. You get an immediate response: when you water something you can see the difference in an hour, and when you weed then something new can grow there. (Though I've learned that many of the weeds are edible and nurturing too.)

When I walk out my door every morning and see the big trees on my street, I compliment God about the day I've been given: "Good one, Lord. Thank you."

> I realized it for the first time in my life: there is nothing but mystery in the world, how it hides behind the fabric of our poor, browbeat days, shining brightly, and we don't even know it.
>
> SUE MONK KIDD, THE SECRET LIFE OF BEES

Camas Lilies

by Lynn Unger

Consider the lilies of the field,
the blue banks of camas opening
into acres of sky along the road.
Would the longing to lie down
and be washed by that beauty
abate if you knew their usefulness,
how the natives ground their bulbs
for flour, how the settlers' hogs
uprooted them, grunting in gleeful
oblivion as the flowers fell?
And you—what of your rushed
and useful life? Imagine setting it all down—
papers, plans, appointments, everything—
leaving only a note: "Gone
to the fields to be lovely. Be back
when I'm through with blooming."
Even now, unneeded and uneaten,
the camas lilies gaze out above the grass
from their tender blue eyes.
Even in sleep your life will shine.
Make no mistake. Of course
your work will always matter.
Yet Solomon in all his glory
was not arrayed like one of these.

Spiritual Practice

Mono no aware

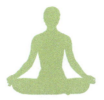

Mono no aware (pronounced ah-whar-eh) is a nearly untranslatable but significant Japanese understanding. The English words that come closest are "the sweet poignancy of things."

Aware means pathos, poignancy, deep feeling, sensitivity, or awareness. Thus, mono no aware has been translated as "the beauty of what is fleeting" or "the 'ahh-ness' of things." In Japan, the cherry blossoms falling in the spring and the brilliant red maple leaves falling in autumn are both times of mono no aware.

Being aware of the impermanence of all things can frighten us, of course. But it can also heighten our appreciation of the beauty and significance of everything around us.

Although this understanding is not as common in the West, many of us with chronic illness have the ability to open to this poignant appreciation of beauty: in the natural world, in the people around us, and in our own lives. In Stephen Levine's book *A Year to Live,* he invites the reader to imagine that we have received a terminal diagnosis and we will die a year from now. How would we choose to live, knowing that? And of course, some of us already have such a diagnosis.

For this spiritual practice, spend some time each day appreciating the world and other people in their impermanence. You could even remind yourself, if you are with someone else, that this person could die tonight, or you could.

Does this practice open your heart to the beauty all around you?

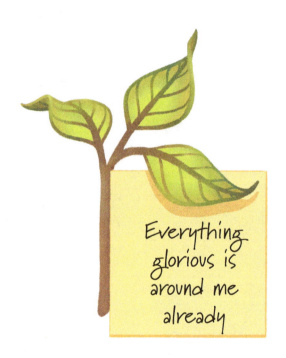

Everything glorious is around me already

All That Is Glorious Around Us

by Barbara Crooker in *Radiance: Poems*

is not, for me, these grand vistas, sublime peaks, mist-filled
overlooks, towering clouds, but doing errands on a day
of driving rain, staying dry inside the silver skin of the car,
160,000 miles, still running just fine. Or later,
sitting in a café warmed by the steam
from white chicken chili, two cups of dark coffee,
watching the red and gold leaves race down the street,
confetti from autumn's bright parade. And I think
of how my mother struggles to breathe, how few good days
she has now, how we never think about the glories
of breath, oxygen cascading down our throats to the lungs,
simple as the journey of water over a rock. It is the nature
of stone / to be satisfied / writes Mary Oliver, It is the nature
of water / to want to be somewhere else, rushing down
a rocky tor or high escarpment, the panoramic landscape
boundless behind it. But everything glorious is around
us already: black and blue graffiti shining in the rain's
bright glaze, the small rainbows of oil on the pavement,
where the last car to park has left its mark on the glistening
street, this radiant world.

Journal Prompts

Where Do I Find Wonder and Beauty?

Wonder then is a force of liberation, It makes sense of what our souls inherently know we were meant for. Every mundane glimpse is salve on a wound, instructions for how to set the bone right again. If you really want to get free, find God on the subway, find God in the soap bubble.

Me? I meet God in the taste of my gramma's chicken, I hear God in the raspy leather of Nina Simone's voice, I see the face of God in the bony teenager bagging my groceries and why shouldn't I? My faith is held together by wonder—by every defined commitment to presence and paying attention.

COLE ARTHUR RILEY, *THIS HERE FLESH*

For this journal prompt, just make a list, as in the quote above. Where do you find wonder? Beauty? Awe? Bliss? Where do you find God, if that language is meaningful for you?

See how many things you can list, from the magnificent to the ordinary. Then notice how you feel.

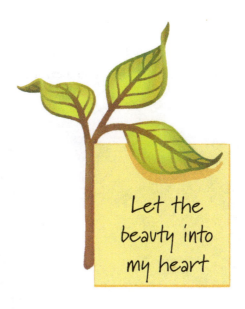

Reflection Questions
Beauty and Bliss

- Share one of the most beautiful experiences of your life, and notice how it feels to talk or write about it.

- What do you notice about how beauty relates to your senses? Do you experience beauty most in hearing, seeing, tasting, smelling, feeling...?

- What gets in your way of fully experiencing beauty?

- What is one thing you could do, within the limits of the life you have, to bring yourself more of an awareness of beauty and wonder?

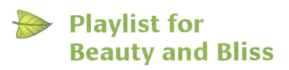

Playlist for Beauty and Bliss

A Thousand Beautiful Things by Annie Lennox

What a Wonderful World by Louis Armstrong, sung by
Playing for Change

A Great Wild Mercy by Carrie Newcomer

Ordinary Magic by Lea Morris

Beautiful Day by U2

For the Beauty of the Earth, words by Folliott Sandford
Pierpoint, music by Conrad Kocher, sung by Audrey Assad

Hallelujah by MaMuse

I Can See Clearly Now by Johnny Nash

How Could Anyone by Shaina Noll

Glorious by MaMuse

Waterfall by Chris Williamson

Morning Has Broken (traditional hymn), sung by
Yusuf/Cat Stevens

15

Play and Joy

When you recover or discover something that nourishes your soul and brings joy, care enough about yourself to make room for it in your life.

Jean Shinoda Bolen

Summer is a time for connecting with joy, playfulness, and a sense of adventure. Whether you are enjoying summer from a bed, balcony, backyard, or the beach, summer is a time to find a balm for your spirit. It can mean cracking a window in the morning to hear birdsong or getting outside to enjoy nature, if that is possible for you. Maybe you can catch up on your favorite author or podcast. You can also delight your tastebuds! Summer is a great time to get fresh produce from local farmers or a garden and enjoy your favorite seasonal foods. Maybe you enjoy getting something cold like ice cream or sorbet or getting into water to cool off from the summer heat.

When we aren't feeling well, the last thing on our minds might be playfulness. Yet play is positive for our spiritual, physical, and mental well-being. Chronic health issues can lead to many limitations on activities or experiences, but there are still ways to find enjoyment and nurture a sense of play. Some people enjoy watching a good comedy or playing games. Others might enjoy coloring books, crossword puzzles, or crafts.

Researcher Barbara Frederickson studies positive emotions like joy and the impact they can have on our lives. She found that joy makes us want to play, expand our curiosity, and connect with others. Through deeply felt experiences of joy, people increase their creativity and resilience. What are some spiritual practices that might help you find joy and a sense of playfulness?

Laughter is a quick way to connect with joy. According to researchers at the Mayo Clinic, laughter really is good medicine: it enhances your intake of oxygen-rich air, stimulates your heart, lungs, and muscles, and increases the endorphins released by your brain. A rollicking laugh fires up and then cools down your stress response, increasing and then decreasing your heart rate and blood pressure.

The resources in this section encourage you to find your inner child, be curious and maybe even blow a few bubbles. Enjoy!

> At the height of laughter, the universe is flung into a kaleidoscope of new possibilities.
>
> JEAN HOUSTON

Claiming the Power of Play and Laughter

Julianne's Story

> Nothing lights up the brain like play.
>
> **Dr. Stuart Brown, *Play Is More Than Fun* TED Talk**

When I was first diagnosed with rheumatoid arthritis, I struggled to understand how to cope with and manage my pain. It was overwhelming, and I felt quite lost. Play and laughter have often been a go-to resource for me, so they seemed to be natural tools to try. I have found, since those early days, that self-care includes nurturing myself with rest, laughter, and play.

When I'm having a rough day and I don't want to get out of bed, I'll try to distract myself with a book, a funny post on social media, or a hopeful news story to get my mind off the pain. Calling a funny friend, watching a lighthearted show, or playing board games or video games can help transport me to a different place.

Sometimes we need to be reminded that there are feelings other than pain and discomfort. We have the right to seek joy, pleasure, and play. Even and especially when we're hurting.

Some people struggle to find time for the joy that might have come easier in younger years. According to play researcher Stuart Brown, remembering our "play history" is an important step in developing our adult experiences of play. Our history gives us insights into what we may find enjoyable in our adult lives. What made you laugh? What types of play did you enjoy the most? Did you have play dates with others? Would a play date at an art studio or trivia night bring out that sense of shared play and joy? Julia

Cameron, who wrote *The Artist's Way*, encourages you to do artist dates with yourself to rekindle your creativity and joy. This can be as simple as swinging on a swing or noticing all the different types of people walking by as you sit on a park bench.

As a child, I used to sit with my grandfather while my mother and grandmother shopped. We would watch people go by and I'd describe my imagined stories of their lives as they passed. "Papa, see that guy? He has three children and lives in a big house by a lake. I bet he fishes all the time." Or, "Papa, see that kid? That kid is lonely, but she has a magic unicorn that tells her secrets every day." Papa would laugh at my stories, and his laughter brought me as much joy as the stories did.

As a little girl, I also had an imaginary spaceship in my closet. I would hide in there for hours and go on space voyages like I saw on Buck Rogers or Star Trek. I glued homemade drawings of computers to the wall and used stickers to create a display screen. I would sometimes put a sleeping bag in there and camp out, with my stuffed animals as my trusty ship's crew.

As an adult, I've tried to embrace that little imaginative girl. I enjoy playing creative characters in games or thinking of strategic ways to get out of sticky situations. I also love to dress up for Renaissance festivals and Halloween, where I can play a character for the day or evening. My family and I have also hosted pirate-themed game parties, where we dress up, decorate the house, and have a blast. I use playful imagination in writing science fiction or fantasy stories, and even in my Sunday sermons for my Unitarian Universalist congregation.

Whether it is an artist date or playing pickleball with friends, we are wired with a need for joy, imagination, and play. My books, writing, and games have helped me through so many hard times and into a better place.

To truly laugh, you must be able to take your pain, and play with it.

CHARLIE CHAPLAIN

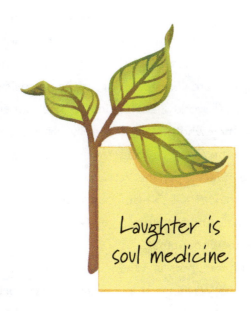

Enjoy Your Life, Don't Let It Stop You

Kathleen's Story

I'm seventy-eight years old. I feel young at heart, but I get treated as if I'm an old lady. And that's shocking to me, like when I go to a counter at the airport and they ask me, "Do you want a wheelchair?"

I have Parkinson's, but I can still walk and my balance is good, so I think of myself as an agile person. Yet when I try to drink from a glass of water, I can't get the glass up to my mouth without splashing everywhere. It's embarrassing to ask for help, but I'm learning to do that rather than make a mess. People have been wonderful in helping me when I ask, but that's hard on my ego.

I transitioned from male to female in 1999. I have not found a relationship since I transitioned. That's difficult for me. Fortunately, my son and his wife are very accepting, but they are literally on the other side of the world. I feel fortunate, since so many trans people have lost their whole family. My family was accepting. And I'm a graduate of the Air Force Academy and even the Air Force Academy has been very accepting. Yet I look back and realize there hasn't been a day since I was three or four years old when I wasn't thinking about male and female and gender. My life would have been very different without that.

I'm an adventurous person. When I was in the second grade we lived in Bellevue, Washington, and I walked to school through the rainforest. I was forbidden to cross a particular road, but mom didn't say anything about crawling through the drainage pipe that went under the road! My best friend and I crawled through the pipe and explored the swamp on the other side and got lost. We were way overdue home and mom found us walking along the roadside, all wet. So exploring new places has been part of my modus operandi for a long time.

I get energy from being around other people and from nature. And I'm still traveling. I just went to Turkey for sixteen days and had a wonderful time, and four weeks later I went to Spain to see my son and daughter-in-law. I love exploring new places and meeting new people, trying brand new foods and learning about the political situation in the places I visit. I try not to take unnecessary risks, but I do take risks. The risk is not the first thing that comes to mind when I'm planning a trip; it's not the limiting factor. I was raised differently from my sisters, who were told they needed to be careful because they were girls.

After I was diagnosed with Parkinson's I wanted to get into a drug trial, but that has been frustrating. I would much rather be in a trial and die doing something useful than just take the current medications. I'm still hoping to get in one. That's an adventure in a totally different way, but it's a way to contribute. That's something that I would like to do even if that shortens my remaining time. I did a lot of work in Haiti, and I would like to get back there too.

If I meet someone newly diagnosed with Parkinson's, I tell them to exercise and to enjoy life. Don't let it stop you and don't stop doing what you love because you've got Parkinson's.

Light De Light

by Peter Levitt

When I lived in San Francisco in 1967 one of our hippie roommates put a little note below the light switch in the kitchen. Simple enough, it said Light De Light.

I've never forgotten that, clearly, or the sweet, playful intention of his writing that gave me that pleasure. That delight.

We think of play as something children do and need, but let's look more closely. As we age, those of us lucky enough to do so, we need play easily as much as when we were children. Possibly more? It keeps the grunge of how the world can grind us down from sticking to our spirit. At the very least. It nourishes love and the imagination. And so much more. It can connect us with others, like my buddy writing Light De Light. He didn't need to write that for himself; he already had the thought. So he wrote it for the rest of us. Bodhisattva in action. And here I am all these years later passing it on to you.

One day someone asked me how I could be happy in such a terrible world. Wasn't I paying attention? I answered simply: It's an obligation. I was thinking about how when people use the word "mitzvah" to mean a good deed, it often is used to mean something special, something extra. But that's not what mitzvah means. A mitzvah is an obligation. We must do it, we are obliged to do it, some act that might be seen as special or extra, but that is not.

For me, being happy in our difficult world is the same. And I don't mean artificial pasty-smile happy; I mean happy for real, because the world is so much more than difficult. I'm sure you've noticed.

And play can be part of that, after all. Part of happy, part of delight, or lighting de light. It doesn't have to be a big deal, either. Simple things. This morning, because like everyone I am multi-minded, my silly mind imagined someone asking me how I would describe my wife and me, our relationship. Shirley comes from a good solid Scottish root, so in my imaginary conversation I said, quick as a whippet, Our relationship? Oh, A Lass and a Lack. And when I thought it, or heard it in my silly mind, it made me happy. So playful. And because it made me happy, when I saw Shirley a little later, I told her about this conversation, and it made her laugh, before saying, You're so silly. So there it is. A bit of play that comes under the heading of Light De Light. Quick as an imagination, a sentence. Spot on as your Uncle Bob.

Please play. Play more. It not only honors life as it is and can be, its reach can travel decades, miles, minds, hearts, generations, forevers. And it's fun.

Smiles, giggles or chuckles are like sips of water.
To feel nourished inside and out, I try to get in as
many tears-streaming, tummy-aching, mess-up-
your-makeup, rip-snorting laughs as I can every day.
CARMEN AMBROSIO, *LIFE CONTINUES*

Joy

by Terri Dennehy in *Becoming*

I have been wondering
what the morning glories
know. Is it envy
that compels these vines
to strangle other flowers
arising in their path?

Or perhaps self-preservation,
to climb these walls, forsaking
humbler beings, winding
greedy stems around the trellis
in their hungry pursuit of light.

Still, every morning,
basking in their spiral shadows,
I want to believe it is something more

this fevered yearning
to open purple flowers,
yield bold-throated *Glorias*
to the sun,
and in the blaze of afternoon
curl petals softly into shyness.

PLAY AND JOY

And every morning, I plead
with the dew-moist buds
to know their secret joy:
to open and close without holding,
to surrender all to light,
to sing
I am completely yours
over and over again.

The Stars Are Dancing

by Om Prakash in *Becoming: A Spiritual Guide for Navigating Adulthood*

The stars are dancing tonight,
while the moon sits in her golden hammock,
swaying back and forth
to the rhythm of celestial voices.

The Beloved is full of rapture,
dancing worlds and stars into being,
drunk with the wine of passion
and filling the heavens with song.

Do not sit alone in the dark
While creation sings three-part harmony.
Dance, my friends.
Dance wildly,
sing joyfully,
fill your heart with the beauty of the Beloved
as the Beloved turns your soul to light.

From *The Book of Joy: Lasting Happiness in a Changing World*

by the Dalai Lama and Desmond Tutu
with Douglas Carlton Abrams

One of the most stunning aspects of the week was how much of it was spent laughing. At times the Dalai Lama and the Archbishop seemed to be as much a comedy duo as two venerable spiritual teachers. It is their ability to joke, and laugh, and poke fun at the ordinary pieties that so righteously violates expectation. When a Dalai Lama and an Archbishop walk into a bar, you don't expect them to be the ones cracking the jokes. . . .

It was clear that humor was central to their joyful way of being, but why was laughter so central?

"I worked with a Mexican shaman once," I said, introducing the topic. "He said that laughing and crying are the same thing—laughing just feels better. It's clear that laughter is central to the way that you are in the world. And the Archbishop was just saying, Your Holiness, that you laugh at something that could ordinarily be a source of anguish."

"That's right. That's right."

"Can you tell us about the role of laughter and humor in the cultivation of joy?"

"It is much better when there is not too much seriousness," the Dalai Lama responded. "Laughter, joking is much better. Then we can be completely relaxed. I met some scientists in Japan, and they explained that wholehearted laughter—not artificial laughter—is very good for your heart and your health in general." When he said "artificial laughter," he pretended to smile and forced a chuckle. He was making a connection between wholehearted laughter and a warm heart, which he had already said was the key to happiness.

Spiritual Practice

Play

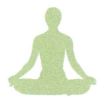

In this spiritual practice, you are invited to find the silly and find your inner trickster and fool. Permit yourself to break loose and put down your worries for this time. Allow yourself to connect to playfulness and a spirit of adventure.

Wes Nisker has written a book about the wisdom that comes to us through tricksters and holy fools called *The Essential Crazy Wisdom*. He says that the fool is the "most potent of the archetypes" and that there are two kinds of fools: "the foolish fool and the great fool." The foolish are inept and silly. They are the ones we see "every day when we look into the mirror or walk down the street." Great fools, on the other hand, are very rare. They invite us into playful wisdom and are "wise beyond ordinary understanding."

For this spiritual practice, set aside at least thirty minutes. What is a joyful, playful activity that you normally don't get to do? Take a chance to do something that might feel risky or foolish. Wear bunny ears to the store or around the house, play a game from childhood, or color in a coloring book. The spiritual practice of play invites us to experience joy and laughter. It is a great resource to manage pain and distract from the challenges of chronic illness.

From *The More or Less Definitive Guide to Self-Care*

by Anna Borges

When was the last time you laughed so hard that your lungs rattled against your ribcage? That you had so much fun you lost track of time? That you weren't afraid of looking stupid? Maybe it's been a while. Maybe it feels out of the question, with everything going on. Maybe you just think you're too old.

The thing is, you can be childlike without being childish, so make time to play anyway. It might look different now than it did when you were a child, but the intention can be the same. See if you can't transport yourself back to that feeling of free-spiritedness. Play for the sake of it, with no purpose or ulterior motive other than to open yourself up to joy and to shake the dust off the shelves in your heart to make more room for the beautiful, wonderful, marvelous things your life has to offer. When we're surrounded by darkness, playfulness is an act of resistance. Wield positivity like a weapon and have fun doing it. If you have to play with your kids (or a friend's kid! or a niece or nephew!) to reawaken some childlike wonder in yourself, do it. The parents would probably appreciate a babysitter.

Journal Prompts

Play

We don't stop playing because we grow old; we
grow old because we stop playing.

GEORGE BERNARD SHAW

- What are times that playfulness has helped you cope with chronic illness?

- Do you have favorite games or ways that you engage in play on a regular basis?

- What is a playful approach that you could take to tasks or activities where you need more joy?

- Describe a memory where play made a difference in your well-being.

Like a welcome summer rain, humor may suddenly
cleanse and cool the earth, the air and you.

LANGSTON HUGHES

Reflection Questions

Play and Joy

- What did your family, friends, or faith tradition teach you about joy, laughter, and play? What kind of play was important to you in early life? How might that be important now?

- Why is play valuable?

- What role do play and laughter have in your daily life? How could laughter and play support your healing journey?

Can you remember the last time you experienced laughter or joy? Whether it was thanks to silly memes or a comedy show, give yourself credit for making time for the lighter side of life.

Give yourself a gold leaf!

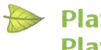 ## Playlist for
Play and Joy

Freedom by John Batiste

Don't Stop Me Now by Queen

Girls Just Want to Have Fun by Cyndi Lauper

I Wanna Dance with Somebody by Whitney Houston

Footloose by Kenny Loggins

Feeling Good by Nina Simone

Cover Me in Sunshine by Pink and Willow Sage Hart

Walking on Sunshine by Katrina and the Waves

New Shoes by Paoli Nutini

It Don't Mean a Thing (If It Ain't Got That Swing)
by Duke Ellington

16
Acceptance

Acceptance is the end of our argument with reality.

Mary Pipher

We deliberately chose "acceptance" as the last chapter in this book. Acceptance is a tricky word: we can judge ourselves for not having it or fool ourselves into thinking we do. Clenching one's teeth in endurance is not acceptance, though on the surface it might seem to be. Passive resignation is not acceptance. Pretending everything is all right when it's not is not acceptance.

Nor is acceptance necessarily about accepting that your current condition is just "how it is" and giving up on getting better, though for some people, with conditions that are not likely to change, coming to terms with not getting better can be an essential form of acceptance. Even then, it is possible to heal on levels other than the physical; one can also heal emotionally and spiritually.

Acceptance is an active process. As the Zen teacher Darlene Cohen writes in *Turning Suffering Inside Out*, "Truly accepting pain is not at all like passive resignation. Rather, it is active engagement with life in its most intimate sense."

Acceptance is also not static: the degree to which we can engage with our life and our physical condition will vary from day to day and even hour to hour. It is not a state we reach at the top of some sort of spiritual pinnacle and then hang out on, cool as a cucumber.

Acceptance is a big space that can—and likely will—include at some point all the difficulties described earlier in this book: grief, anger, pain, isolation, fear, and all the rest. What does that mean? Just as we can compassionately accept a friend's grief or anger, it is possible to accept our own. This is sometimes called *radical acceptance*. This term was introduced by the psychologist Marsha Linehan, who writes, "Radical acceptance rests on letting go of the illusion of control and a willingness to notice and accept things as they are right now, without judging. [It is a] complete and total openness to the facts of reality as they are."

There is a famous poem by the Sufi poet and mystic Rumi, as translated by Coleman Barkes, that begins: "This being human is a guest house. Every morning a new arrival. Welcome and entertain them all! Even if they are a crowd of sorrows . . ." This is the spirit of radical acceptance.

My happiness grows in direct proportion to my acceptance, and in inverse proportion to my expectations.

MICHAEL J. FOX

Can I Love the Life I Have?

Florence's Story

Earlier this summer I was struck by the realization that it has been exactly twenty-five years that chronic illness has been powerfully shaping my life. That's a quarter of a century. In fact, my first autoimmune illness began in the *last century*. If illness was a child, they'd be out of the house at this age (I hope!) and working somewhere, renting an apartment. Instead, chronic illness lives in this body: sometimes at the wheel of the car and determining the direction of my life, sometimes sitting in the back seat, temporarily quiescent, like a child looking out the window.

Speaking of driving, last summer I drove from the Midwest out to Colorado, California, and the Pacific Northwest and back again, leading retreats, guest preaching at several Unitarian Universalist congregations, and giving dharma talks in various Zen communities. For most of the last twenty-five years I would not have been capable of such a trip. Old friends I saw on the journey asked about my health, and I answered honestly: "I'm doing really well, better than I've been for the last four years, but I never take this for granted. I know it all could change tomorrow, and I'm grateful for what I have today." Luckily my health remained strong for the duration of the trip. I may even be in a remission from rheumatoid arthritis—for now.

There is tremendous humility in living a life so marked by chronic illness. I've had to learn to respond with compassion to the requests of the body, to treat the body as a partner rather than an enemy. This is most true when the lights go dark and we are once again whirling into the territory of pain and weakness. It's easy to fight and resist, but I've learned the hard way how resistance increases the suffering. Instead there has to be a kind of surrender. The body is firmly in the lead, and my job is to follow it. That's what this partner has taught me.

I now recognize that pride is a big part of my personality. There's nothing like a good illness to help you release a little excess pride. Proud of your dependability? Illness makes you undependable. Proud of your self-sufficiency? Illness forces you to ask for help. Proud of your career? Illness may very well undermine whatever career you have.

We're taught in Buddhism that the degree of suffering is directly related to the degree of holding on. Despite this teaching, most of us don't let go of anything very easily. Illness, like a new puppy who chews anything and everything in sight, helps us get rid of things we thought we needed but really didn't. Somehow, miraculously, every time I lose some part of my self-image, something fresh and beautiful comes my way. Because of this illness, I'm way less impressive, but there's more room for grace.

In some circles, we are told that illness is a gift. I have found that the "gifts" of being sick are far more complicated than that. I can remember snarling at someone, years ago, when they suggested that my illness might be a gift. Folks, a word of advice here: however much you may want to, refrain from making this suggestion to a sick person. They won't thank you. Finding the gift of illness can only come from some genuine place far within. From without, it feels like a way of minimizing the tremendous suffering of the person who is sick.

I couldn't call it a gift, not for years. It felt like a curse, actually, something entirely undeserved, unwarranted, and unnecessary. I have to say that it still feels like a curse some days, but there are gifts there too. And the greatest and hardest gift? The visceral, direct knowledge that life is not limitless, that tomorrow is completely unknown, and that, literally, there is no time to waste.

So, illness is a dance, an admonition, a curse, a blessing, the divine chosen deity. I would not wish it on anyone: it's a rough, cruel road. Nonetheless, here I am. How can I not bow down to it? It has humbled me and stripped me bare; it has given me my true life.

Acceptance has meant to me, over these years, seeing both my times of health and my times of fatigue and pain as the life I have. I now see this particular life as a long dance with illness, though it wasn't the dance I would have chosen. Nonetheless it has led me in life-giving directions.

I am grateful for my times of relative well-being over these twenty-five years, though I never take them for granted. I know that physical well-being, like everything else in life, is impermanent, maybe especially impermanent in my case. And I allow myself grief when life is harder. But I have also learned that there can be plenty of joy, plenty of beauty, plenty of spiritual deepening even then. In writing this book, Julianne and I have hoped to give you a taste of these possibilities, and resources, for your own journey through chronic illness or pain.

The world that opened to me through engaging the physical suffering and mental anguish caused by my disease has turned out to be inexpressibly rich. Because if we can engage with our suffering—connect with it, dance with it, tease it, coax it, curse it, as well as trying to change it, just consider it our lives, experience it as our lives, the only lives we have—it changes the quality of that suffering. It's not just our suffering; it's everything.

DARLENE COHEN, *Turning Suffering Inside Out*

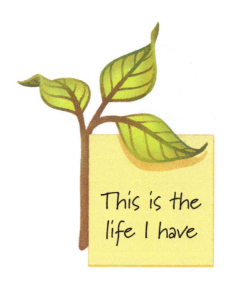

People ask me, "Have you tried yoga? Kombucha? This special water?" And I don't have the energy to explain that yes, I've tried them. I've tried crystals and healing drum circles and prayer and everything. What I want to try is acceptance. I want to see what happens if I can simply accept myself for who I am: battered, broken, hoping for relief, still enduring somehow.

I will still take a cure if it's presented to me, but I am so tired of trying to bargain with the universe for some kind of cure. The price is simply too high to live chasing cures, because in doing so, I'm missing living my life.

I know only that in chasing to achieve the person I once was, I will miss the person I have become.

LIZ MOORE, "I'M TIRED OF CHASING A CURE," IN *DISABILITY VISIBILITY*

From "Acceptance Is Not Passive; It's the Path to Peace"

by Shunya Anding

Diagnosed with lupus, an autoimmune disease, and a future of chronic pain or worse, I had to give up the impressive job, the active social life, and the self-image that had all propped me up in the world. And then what was left?

Instinctively, I wanted to go back to the way things were, to repatch it all back together again. Fortunately, I inherently felt the impossibility of all of that, and so the work began.

I started taking a meditation class and then a Buddhist practice, and one day sitting silently, feeling my body breathing, listening inwardly to what was there, the hard, guarding shell around my heart broke. I had to accept there was no going back to normal, there was only being with what is and opening to where that might lead. . . .

Allowing myself to actually be the way I felt, without the weight of someone else's expectations, was the beginning of moving toward physical and emotional health.

Rilke writes, "Gravity is like an ocean current that takes hold of even the strangest thing and pulls it toward the earth. We need to patiently trust our heaviness—even a bird must do this before it can fly."

Trusting that the earth will support all of our weight, all of our heaviness, the physical pain and the mental anguish too, brings us to a place of feeling grounded, a place that's ready to respond with wisdom and compassion, though this does take practice.

Healing into Whatever's Next

Ellen's Story

I am a 73-year-old white woman, a musician and singer-songwriter. I was raised Catholic, but when I was thirteen, I had a powerful personal mystical experience, and the message was that it was not for me to follow a particular religion, but it was to find my own path.

In 2021, I started being dizzy a lot, losing my balance and having headaches. I had had Covid and I went to doctors and they kept saying, "It's probably just long Covid." And then in the middle of the night, in March of 2022, I remembered that my brother Michael and my favorite uncle Gene had both died of glioblastomas back in the 1980s. And so I talked to my nurse and she ordered a CT scan.

On April 11th, 2022, a friend drove me to get the scan. On the way home I got a message saying, "You have a brain tumor," and they wanted me at the hospital right away. I remember just sitting there and thinking, "Okay, I guess we all at some point get something, have to face something." And I thought, "Am I supposed to be kind of miserable or afraid or something?" Literally, I felt like I tried those on. And I thought, "Those don't suit me. That's not how I want to spend whatever time I have left." And I thought, "This is really interesting. I've never had a brain tumor before." And I made a very conscious choice at that point to be as curious, to find it as interesting as possible, and also to be as loving as possible. I didn't even know what that meant. And I still don't. I mean, what the heck is love? I couldn't really define it.

I felt like this was a chance for me to be who I really am and be connected and not put my pain on anybody else. And I also realized that for me, humor was in there too. Some of the doctors didn't quite get my humor, but maybe eventually they did.

After we got the news, I went to the hospital that night, which is quite a drive from the rural area where I live. I met with the neurosurgeon the next morning, and he told me, "I don't see you getting any better without surgery." And he told me that the tumor was sitting on my cerebellum and brainstem. At that time they didn't know if it was cancerous or benign (it was benign).

I remember sliding into the MRI before the surgery and talking to my tumor and thanking it. I said, "Thank you for being there, for showing me what you need to let me know. You're not going to be here after tomorrow, and I bless you on your journey." The poor little tumor, where did it go? Part of me is somewhere else.

The whole experience of the surgery and recovery was one of the most profound experiences of my life. And I felt that way for quite a while afterwards. I knew I was deeply held by those I'd touched—known and unknown—and by life itself. One dear friend asked, "So is it really recovery? Are you going back to what you were?" And I said, "No, I don't think so. It's healing into whatever's next."

Spiritual Practice
The Path to Peace

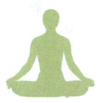

None of us can escape disappointment and sorrow in life. They come with the territory. They're part of the human condition, largely because we don't control a good portion of what happens to us. If there's no escaping our measure of disappointment and sorrow, then the path to peace and well-being must lie in learning to open our hearts and minds to embrace whatever life is serving up at the moment. This is a mindfulness practice—mindfulness infused with compassion for ourselves.

TONI BERNHARD, *HOW TO LIVE WELL WITH CHRONIC PAIN AND ILLNESS*

Find a large, soft blanket or shawl and wrap yourself up in it, either sitting or lying down. Feel yourself held and embraced as you breathe.

Imagine that your mind and heart are expanding beyond the boundaries of your body, filling the room around you, or maybe even out into the sky, and that there is enough room for all of you and everything you feel in that big space.

Keeping that sense of expansion, bring to mind your current sorrows and disappointments. Perhaps you can even imagine them outside you, but within your expanded heart and mind. What do they look like?

Although it may be difficult, can you offer compassion and kindness to these sorrows? To these guests in the guesthouse of being human? If tears come, welcome them too.

When you're ready, come back to the feeling of being held. End with a hand on your heart and a blessing for yourself, whatever comes to mind.

From *Let the Whole Thundering World Come Home: A Memoir*

by Natalie Goldberg

For me this wasn't war, something to fight. Disease was another aspect of human life. Could I be in the middle of it, not so much be victorious but actually flower, become more tender, more inside human understanding? Could it open love? And reflection? Could I stand inside the storm, be drenched and endure, whether into life or into death? . . .

This is my one heavenly life. This afternoon. This Thursday. This sun on the pale dirt and the cottonwood green leaves. This blue mesa in the distance, this gutsy temporary life lived as the Buddha taught—with gusto.

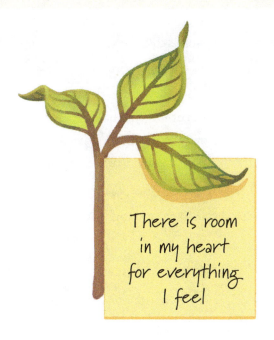

There is room in my heart for everything I feel

Journal Prompts
Essential Goodness

The Buddha taught that this human birth is a precious gift because it gives us the opportunity to realize the love and awareness that are our true nature. As the Dalai Lama pointed out.... we all have Buddha nature. Spiritual awakening is the process of recognizing our essential goodness, our natural wisdom and compassion.... The very nature of our heart is to care.

TARA BRACH

- Name a few examples of how you have expressed goodness, wisdom, or compassion over the course of your life. Since this is a private place, you don't have to worry that you are tooting your own horn.

- Who or what do you care about right now? How do you express that caring?

- Does this human birth feel like a precious gift? Why or why not?

- How do you live well even with chronic pain or illness? Can you list ten ways you live well?

Reflection Questions

Acceptance

- What are some of your top ten ways of living well even while sick?

- What does acceptance mean to you at this moment?

- Who are the people who support you?

- What gifts, if any, have come from being sick?

Can you, just for a moment, accept all of who you are right now, warts and all?

Give yourself a gold leaf!

Playlist for Acceptance

Acceptance by Frankie Orella

Broken and Beautiful by Kelly Clarkson

Little Wonders by Rob Thomas

Beautiful by Austin Plaine

I Rise by Madonna

Stand in the Light by Jordan Smith

Rise by Eddie Vedder

Every Little Bit of It by Carrie Newcomer

It's OK by Nightbirde

GUIDED MEDITATIONS

All guided meditations are available on the companion website, tend-to-your-spirit.info/meditations.

FALL

A Guided Meditation on Spaciousness to Ease Pain

With thanks to Les Fehmi and his book *Dissolving Pain*

Feel your whole body sitting on a chair or a cushion. You don't need to be in a special position for this meditation, although I suggest sitting with your eyes closed.

Feel your whole body here with whatever the experiences are of the body at this moment.

And then feel or sense the space around the body, the space in the room, the room held in the space beyond the room, the sky above.

Really connect with the sensations or awareness of the space all around us all the time.

And as you breathe, realize that you're breathing in air from the space around you, and you're releasing air into the space around you.

Now, bring your attention to a part of your body where there is no discomfort. This might be your hands, for instance. Just feel your hands. Perhaps they're in your lap. Perhaps they're in contact with each other. Just feel your hands here.

Now, whatever sensations may be there, narrow down to a small area within the area you have chosen—perhaps your thumb, your left thumb—and feel whatever sensations may be there in your thumb. There might be energy or warmth, coolness or pressure, whatever it is that you feel.

(And again, if you're choosing a different part of your body, you can just do this practice in another part of the body.)

And then in your imagination, go inside your thumb. This thumb that is surrounded by space, just as your whole body is surrounded by space. And especially if our eyes are closed, there's no really obvious division between inside and outside.

So if you bring your attention to that cloud of sensations in the thumb, imagine going inside the thumb and feeling the space that is actually within every cell, every atom. There's vast space within atoms. We think that we're solid, but in reality, we are mostly space.

See if you can connect with the sense of space inside one of your thumbs. And then expand that sense of both the space inside and the space outside, and that there's really no sharp division between them, to the whole area of your hands.

Feel the spaciousness inside your hands and then expand that sense of spaciousness throughout the body.

So, with your eyes closed, feel that cloud of sensations in the body.

Sometimes I say it's like a cloud of butterflies that are all moving in the same direction. No sharp division between inside and outside. And just rest in this spacious space of the body.

Perhaps there is a place within the body where there is discomfort or perhaps full-on pain. As gently as possible, and only when you really feel ready, go to the edge of that sensation—not to the middle, but to the edge, to the area around the sensation—and connect with the feeling of space. No matter how contracted that area of our body might be, no matter how much we may feel contracted within in response.

And if you have multiple areas, just choose one for this and just go to the edge of the discomfort. Just rest your awareness there.

Pain has a way of drawing the attention into it. So I just invite you again, stay at the edge and feel the spaciousness there.

Feel all the space that exists between cell and cell between atom and atom, and within atoms.

And if you can stay present with that feeling of the edge of discomfort, you can enter more deeply into the area that is uncomfortable in your body. Again, very gently, not forcing anything.

If it's only just for a moment that you can be present with that area, please take care of yourself, but feel the space even within the discomfort.

Notice that even with whatever is there, there is space in between the sensations, and there is of course space all around the body.

Let the sensations be dissolved within that great spaciousness within and without.

And then come back to the sensation of the whole body here, the cloud again of what we feel with our eyes closed and the space around and within us.

And just rest there until you are ready to open your eyes.

WINTER

A Guided Meditation on Comfort and Pleasure

For this guided meditation on comfort and pleasure, find the most comfortable position in which to experience this meditation.

Perhaps it's lying down or sitting in a recliner, or maybe even lying on the grass in your backyard. Whatever truly gives you comfort.

Make sure that the temperature is comfortable for you and see if you need to have a blanket over you or to change your clothing in some way.

Again, the idea is to find the most comfortable position.

Once you've found a position and are resting there, really allow your bones and muscles and ligaments to rest, to be supported by whatever you are sitting or lying down upon.

From this place of comfort, we will explore each of the senses. The intention here is to see if you can find comfort or pleasure in each of the senses.

Let's begin with feeling and touch. Perhaps the very feeling of resting comfortably evokes pleasure, or perhaps touching something nearby is pleasurable: a cat curled in your lap or the feeling of the blanket around you.

Just notice how it is to connect with pleasure and comfort as you rest.

If there is nothing nearby that is pleasurable, find something in your house that is nice to hold or touch. Notice how your body responds.

Now notice with your ears if there's any sound in your environment that is pleasurable.

Perhaps you have soft music on, or there's birdsong outside your window, or maybe even the silence has a kind of pleasure. Just enjoy whatever may be true.

If there isn't any overtly pleasurable sound, just notice what is neutral.

If your eyes have been closed, open your eyes and look around the space that you're in and see if there's something that brings pleasure to your eyes.

Maybe it's a vase of flowers, or a painting on your wall, or the view out your window. Really savor and fully experience that pleasure.

For the next two senses, you might want to close your eyes.

Imagine your very favorite food, some kind of food that is truly a comfort food for you.

As much as you can, imagine the experience of tasting that food, really letting yourself revel in the pleasure of your favorite food.

Now bring to mind in your imagination the most wonderful smell, the smell that gives you the greatest of pleasures.

Maybe it's the smell of something cooking on the stove or baking in the oven. Maybe it's the smell of a particular flower. Maybe it's the smell of a beloved person's perfume or cologne.

Bring that smell to mind. Again, let yourself roll around in it with pleasure.

And after you have explored all your five senses, come back to the restfulness of where you are at the moment.

Notice if your body or mind or spirit feels a little different after this meditation on pleasure and comfort.

SPRING

A Guided Meditation on Change

This is a guided meditation on being aware of changes from moment to moment. You can do this meditation in a seated or lying down position or even walking—whatever feels right to you. If you want, you can play some gentle music as you do this meditation.

Begin by being aware of your whole body, whatever it feels like at the moment.

Next, bring attention to the breath.

Notice how it feels to breathe in: the way the beginning of the breath feels, the deepening of the breath, and then the natural turn toward the outbreath and the feeling—the actual, physical feeling—of the outbreath and the pause before the next inbreath, wherever you feel it most vividly in your body.

Spend a few moments just breathing in and out and noticing the changes.

One of the most powerful ways to be aware of change is through the medium of sound and hearing. So open up your ears really wide and just notice what comes in.

Perhaps there's silence, and then a car goes by and the car gets louder. The sound changes and then fades away.

Maybe the wind comes up and you hear the rustling of leaves. That changes and then diminishes.

Or if you are listening to music, there is the change in tone and in volume. Music, of course, would not exist without change.

And with each change, another moment of life has also changed and has passed.

See if you can have a feeling of curiosity and openness about these changes that are occurring moment by moment.

Spend a few minutes really listening to the world around you as it changes. You might notice that you like some sounds and other sounds are not so pleasant. So not only is the sound changing, but so are you.

Maybe as you do this meditation thoughts come up in your mind: your to-do list or a memory.

Notice how the thoughts appear and have a certain span of time, and then as you pay attention may disappear as well.

If you have some discomfort in the body, you can bring your gentle attention to the discomfort and see if you notice any changes as you pay attention. Please only do this with a mild discomfort, not an overwhelming one.

Even areas of discomfort in the body, if we pay attention, are often changing subtly moment by moment.

We live in a constant sea of change, like the waves on the beach, like the ocean itself, and our body as well is always changing.

This meditation can be a powerful way to begin a longer period of meditation, or as we're walking (without listening to a podcast!), to just notice all the changes: the changes in our vision, in our hearing, in our sensations, in every part of our experience.

Change can be frightening, but it can also bring new experiences and new possibilities.

When you're ready, gently come out of this meditation back into the realm of moment-by-moment life.

SUMMER

A Guided Meditation on Beauty

This meditation can either be done as a seeing meditation or a hearing meditation, depending on what works best for you and your body.

As a seeing meditation, sit outside in a place you find beautiful, or sit by a window facing out.

Begin with your eyes closed.

Start by grounding and settling yourself, feeling your feet on the ground, your breath, your body.

Take as long as you need to feel settled, and when you're ready, open your eyes and let them take in what you see.

Often we judge what we are seeing. In this case, just focus on the positive in what you see.

Let your eyes be drawn to what is most beautiful around you. Let it be as it is, without needing to change it.

Look more and more deeply. Let your eyes rest and be filled by what is beautiful.

If thoughts begin to come up, keep returning to just seeing. Let yourself savor what you see.

Stay with what you see for several minutes. Let yourself fully appreciate. If gratitude arises, let that be part of your experience.

Once you feel saturated with the experience of the beauty you were focused on, choose something else in your visual field, or adjust your position to see something else that is also beautiful.

Once again, focus on the positive, without needing to change it.

Look more and more deeply. Let yourself savor what you see for several minutes.

If you feel comfortable doing so and are able, you could slowly move around the area, looking more closely at things that you are drawn toward. Really look at them, repeating the practice as long as you want.

When you are ready, return and close your eyes again.

Let the beauty you have seen fill your spirit. Check in with your body and see how you feel now.

***

As a hearing meditation, choose a piece of music that seems beautiful to you, perhaps from one of our playlists, but don't play it yet. You can be sitting or lying down. You might want to use headphones to bring the music close.

Start by grounding and settling yourself, feeling your breath and your body.

Take as long as you need to feel settled, and when you're ready, turn on the music. Keep your eyes closed for this meditation.

Often we judge what we are hearing. In this case, just focus on the positive in what you hear. Let it be as it is, without needing to change it.

Listen more and more deeply. Let your mind rest and be filled by what is beautiful.

If thoughts begin to come up, keep returning to just hearing. Let yourself savor what you hear.

Listen for several minutes. Let yourself fully appreciate. If gratitude arises, let that be part of your experience.

If you want, you could choose another piece of music.

Continue until you feel saturated and then allow silence.

Let the beauty you have heard fill your spirit. Check in with your body and see how you feel now.

USING THIS BOOK IN SMALL GROUPS

Chronic illness or chronic pain can be overwhelming and isolating, and having support on the journey can make all the difference. The small discussion groups that accompany this book are called Seasons Circles to honor all the seasons that people live through with chronic illness.

Seasons Circles are small groups, usually composed of no more than ten people, that meet to regularly discuss this book and the reflection questions in each chapter. They can help foster supportive relationships for the ups and downs dealing with chronic illness, allowing them to care for each other even outside of the group.

The small group size keeps them flexible and responsive to the needs of their members. They can also offer authentic sharing and closeness that might be unavailable or uncomfortable in larger groups. These circles are built on trust that will hopefully allow their members to share at progressively deeper levels.

Seasons Circles have some things in common with a support group and some things in common with a book group, but they are more structured and focused on the spiritual practices and readings in *Tend to Your Spirit*. Below are some suggestions for how groups might be organized and facilitated. You can decide as a group how members will interact with one another, what the time commitment will be, and the basic logistics of meetings.

Agreements and Facilitation

We recommend beginning a new group by forming agreements that allow space for everyone to talk and deeply listen to one another and reading these agreements at the beginning of each meeting. Creating agreements on how you will gather and treat each other provides a safe space for growth and sharing and creates the conditions for increased trust over time. Here are some sample agreements from our own experience, but feel free to alter these or create your own as a group:

1. We will maintain confidentiality: what is shared here is confidential and will not be shared outside the group without permission of the person who shared.

2. We will make this circle a priority: members will do their best to attend sessions, health permitting.

3. We will communicate changes with each other: members will notify the whole group if they will not be able to attend a session or if they want to leave the group.

4. We will listen respectfully and compassionately to each other, by not interrupting, judging, or giving advice, unless requested.

It's good to have a facilitator, although this role can rotate. The job of the facilitator is to support an appropriate level of sharing, allowing all to feel comfortable to participate in the group.

Logistics

Small discussion groups allow people to connect with one another in meaningful ways amidst the hustle and bustle of modern life. Seasons Circles do a similar thing—they provide for support around the challenges of living with chronic illness. At each meeting, Circle participants have the opportunity to check in and let others who care about them know what's going on in their lives. Below are some questions to ask as you organize your Season Circle:

- How do we want to organize our group? Will there be one leader or will we take turns with organizing and facilitating?

- How often do we want to meet (weekly? monthly?), for how long, and in what location? Online or in person? (Online will be more accessible for those who are housebound.)

- Do we want to set the number of meetings at the beginning? There are 16 chapters in the book.

- Will we be open to new members?

- Do we want to have a set agenda for meetings or keep things more organic?

- Do we want to begin with a silent or guided meditation?

Sample Seasons Circle

Opening the Circle
Light a candle, ring a chime, or signify in some way the beginning of your time together.

Facilitator Welcome

The facilitator welcomes everyone to the meeting and covers anything that people need to know for the meeting.

Opening Words

You could use a poem or reading from the chapter or substitute one of your own choosing about the theme of the chapter. The facilitator could choose these words.

Meditation

A time of silence or the sharing of a guided meditation, from the book or from elsewhere.

Check-in

This is a chance for members to briefly share personal updates. You could give each person a set amount of time, since this could go long. For in-person meetings, you may wish to use an object or talking stick to pass to one another for this time.

Chapter Discussion

Start with reflections on a chapter from members and ask if there were any practices or readings that sparked ideas or questions. Members can share from journal writing or other insights.

Reflection Questions

Use the questions to deepen reflection on the chapter topic. You may wish to invite members to bring their own questions to share with the group. Allowing each person to reflect on a question before opening up the discussion will allow quieter members a chance to speak.

Closing Words

You could use a poem, reading, or quote from the chapter or substitute one of your own choosing.

Closing the Circle

Extinguish the candle, ring a chime, or signify in some way that this is the end of your time together.

ACKNOWLEDGMENTS

This book began through connection and caretaking between ministerial colleagues when we were both coming to grips with our new diagnoses with rheumatoid arthritis. We want to thank Mary Benard, publications director at Skinner House Books, for believing in this project; Larisa Hohenboken for their excellent editing and thoughtful suggestions; and Pierce Alquist for her promotional support and championing our book. We also offer appreciation to the artist, Alyssa Alarcón Santo, cover designer, Alex Camlin, and text designer, Tim Holtz. Finally, we want to thank the many people who were willing to be interviewed and who spoke with such honesty and vulnerability. Our individual acknowledgments are below.

Julianne

I want to first thank Florence for companioning me through the early hard times of my illness and through the process of creating this book. Her knowledge, wisdom, and caring friendship have absolutely been the glue that got this book to the finish line. I'd also like to thank my partner, Karl Lepp, my children, Ehren and Kendra Lepp, and my mother-in-law, Eleta Reese, for believing so deeply in me and giving substantial support and space to this project. I am appreciative of my dad, Rev. Bob Libbey, and my sister, Gregg Peake, for their enthusiasm and excitement for this book. Thanks to my mom, Julianne Price, who is no longer with us, but was my first and biggest cheerleader as a writer since I've been writing stories in my spaceship bedroom closet.

Much appreciation to the staff and members of the Unitarian Universalist Congregation in Eau Claire, Wisconsin, for their encouragement and good wishes while I worked on completing the final draft of the book during part of my sabbatical leave. Gratitude to Kris Deehr and Aimee Johnson for their listening and support during check-ins at our weekly staff meetings. Thanks to the encouragement from my chalice circles, memoir group, and long-time coffee ladies.

I want to recognize and thank early readers: Karl Lepp, Gregg Peake, Rev. Bob Libbey, Eleta Reese, and Kristen Gustavson. Thank you to Sue Fulkerson, Bob Nowlan, and Tree Nagle, who have shared such compassion and wisdom about chronic illness. I am so grateful to Adria Madera Acosta, MD, and Erin Spritzer, PA-C, for their excellent support and care at the Mayo Clinic Rheumatology Department in Eau Claire, Wisconsin. I feel so blessed by spiritual support from Rev. Stacy Craig, Rev. Jill Braithwaite, Rev. David Huber, and Rev. Kathy Reid-Walker, and by all I've learned about spiritual practice from Rev. Tandi Rogers and my cohort in Spiritual Direction and Formation at the LIGHT program at Meadville Lombard Seminary. Lastly, my gratitude to the Moms with Rheumatoid Facebook group, which has offered a community of support, knowledge, and empathy.

Florence

I want to thank Julianne for her friendship and for inviting me to be part of this book project, which was truly her vision. I also want to thank her for her steadfastness in the process of collaboratively writing and creating the book, with all its bumps and negotiations, and for the lovely hours in our writing retreats in Iowa and on the coast of Washington—particularly sharing Southern food and drink at the Tokeland Hotel!

Over the last two years I have been leading online classes and groups for people with chronic illness and pain called "Dancing in the Dark Fields" through San Francisco Zen Center. I am deeply grateful to the participants for what they have taught me about courage, sincerity, and vulnerability. It has been a great privilege to witness their journeys, and they gave me many ideas about what was important to include in this book.

I want to thank my late mother, Harriet McNeal, for all she showed me about the possibilities for resilience and joy even at the end of life, and my friends and family, particularly Cristy Wickman, Zoe Darling, Dana Lyons, Dana Velden, Jean La Valley, Mark Grote, Michael Hofmann, Eric Harlow, Kevin Atkins, Sue Moon, Mike Sinn, Sally Taylor, Deborah Caplow, Dorothy Echodu, and others, who have, over many years, supported me, believed in me, and at times gently scolded me. I want to thank my homeopath Stephen King, who never stopped believing that healing is possible, and my brilliant functional medicine doctor, Dr. Kathleen Stienstra.

I have been blessed, for four decades now, with the support of the ancient spiritual practices of Buddhism and Buddhist meditation. I want to offer many bows to my Buddhist teachers: James Baraz, who opened the door of practice for me; Norman Fischer, my primary Zen teacher for many years; Bruce Fortin, my heart teacher who "adopted" me; Jeff Kitzes, both therapist and teacher, who accompanied me through so much; Joan Halifax, who has believed in me as I have grown into a teacher myself; and especially the late Darlene Cohen, who offered such invaluable teachings on living with grace with chronic illness.

RESOURCES

Living with Chronic Illness

The Chronic Illness Workbook: Strategies and Solutions for Taking Back Your Life, by Patricia Fennell

Dancing with Elephants: Mindfulness Training for Those Living with Dementia, Chronic Illness or an Aging Brain, by Jarem Sawatsky

How to Be Sick: A Buddhist-Inspired Guide for the Chronically Ill and Their Caregivers, by Toni Bernhard

How to Live Well with Chronic Pain and Illness: A Mindful Guide, by Toni Bernhard

Illness as Metaphor, by Susan Sontag

In the Kingdom of the Sick: A Social History of Chronic Illness in America, by Laurie Edwards

Incurable Optimist: Living with Illness and Chronic Hope, by Jennifer Cramer-Miller

Life Continues: Facing the Challenges of MS, Menopause & Midlife with Hope, Courage & Humor, by Carmen Ambrosio

Super Sick: Making Peace with Chronic Illness, by Allison Alexander

Surviving and Thriving with an Invisible Chronic Illness: How to Stay Sane and Live One Step Ahead of Your Symptoms, by Ilana Jacqueline

What Doesn't Kill You: A Life with Chronic Illness—Lessons from a Body in Revolt, by Tessa Miller

You Don't Look Sick! Living Well with Invisible Chronic Illness, by Joy H. Selak and Steven S. Overman

Living with Chronic Pain

Arthritis: Stop Suffering, Start Moving, by Darlene Cohen

Dissolving Pain: Simple Brain-Training Exercises for Overcoming Chronic Pain, by Les Fehmi and Jim Robbins

Mindfulness Meditation for Pain Relief: Practices to Reclaim Your Body and Your Life, by Jon Kabat-Zinn

Outsmart Your Pain: Mindfulness and Self-Compassion to Help You Leave Chronic Pain Behind, by Christiane Wolf

Turning Suffering Inside Out: A Zen Approach for Living with Physical and Emotional Pain, by Darlene Cohen

Disability and Disability Rights

Being Heumann: An Unrepentant Memoir of a Disability Rights Activist, by Judith Heumann with Kristen Joiner

A Disability History of the United States, by Kim E. Nielson

Disability Visibility: First-Person Stories from the Twenty-First Century, edited by Alice Wong

Loving Our Own Bones: Disability Wisdom and the Spiritual Subversiveness of Knowing Ourselves Whole, by Julia Watts Belser

Sitting Pretty: The View from My Ordinary Resilient Disabled Body, by Rebekah Taussig

Rest, Sabbath, Play, and Joy

Awakening Joy: 10 Steps That Will Put You on the Road to Real Happiness, by James Baraz and Shoshana Alexander

The Book of Joy: Lasting Happiness in a Changing World, by the Dalai Lama and Desmond Tutu with Douglas Abrams

The Essential Crazy Wisdom, by Wes Nisker

Incantations for Rest: Poems, Meditations, and Other Magic, by Atena O. Danner

Hygge: Unlock the Danish Art of Coziness and Happiness, by Barbara Hayden

The More or Less Definitive Guide to Self-Care, by Anna Borges

Pause, Rest, Be: Stillness Practices for Courage in Times of Change, by Octavia F. Raheem

Rest Is Resistance: A Manifesto, by Tricia Hersey

Sabbath: Finding Rest, Renewal, and Delight in Our Busy Lives, by Wayne Muller

Sacred Rest: Recover Your Life, Renew Your Energy, Restore Your Sanity, by Saundra Dalton-Smith

Wintering: The Power of Rest and Retreat in Difficult Times, by Katherine May

Memoirs About Illness

Beyond the Mailbox: A Life with Chronic Illness, by Pat Gavula

Brittle Joints, by Maria Sweeney

A Burst of Light and Other Essays, by Audre Lorde

The Invisible Kingdom: Reimagining Chronic Illness, by Meghan O'Rourke

Let the Whole Thundering World Come Home: A Memoir, by Natalie Goldberg

My Pancreas Broke But My Life Got Better, by Nagata Kabi

My Soul Showed Up: Finding Hope and Resilience Against All Odds, by Pat Henneberry

. . . surprise I have a chronic illness . . . by Angel L. McKenzie

Strong at the Broken Places: Voices of Illness, a Chorus of Hope by Richard M. Cohen

What's Wrong: Personal Histories of Chronic Pain and Bad Medicine, by Erin Williams

You Don't Look Sick: My Journey with an Invisible Illness, by Kristen Dutkiewicz

Poetry and Literary Prose

Circle of Grace: A Book of Blessings for the Seasons, by Jan Richardson

Consolations: The Solace, Nourishment and Underlying Meaning of Everyday Words, by David Whyte

Radiance: Poems, by Barbara Crooker

Spilling the Light, by Julián Jamaica Soto

Into the Wilderness: A Meditation Manual, by Sarah York

Becoming: A Spiritual Guide for Navigating Adulthood, edited by Kayla Parker

Grief and Dying

Alive Until You're Dead: Notes on the Home Stretch, by Susan Moon

Here After: A Memoir, by Amy Lin

A Hole in the World: Finding Hope in Rituals of Grief and Healing by Amanda Held Opelt

We Were Made for These Times: 10 Lessons for Moving Through Change, Loss, and Disruption, by Kaira Jewel Lingo

The Wild Edge of Sorrow: Rituals of Renewal and the Sacred Work of Grief, by Francis Weller

Who Dies?: An Investigation of Conscious Living and Conscious Dying, by Stephen and Ondrea Levine

A Year to Live: How to Live This Year as If It Were Your Last, by Stephen Levine

Caregiving

The Mindful Caregiver: Finding Ease in the Caregiving Journey, by Nancy L. Kriseman

Spirituality, Meditation, Buddhism

Atlas of the Heart: Mapping Meaningful Connection and the Language of Human Experience, by Brené Brown

Being Bodies: Buddhist Women on the Paradox of Embodiment, edited by Lenore Friedman and Susan Moon

Comfortable with Uncertainty: 108 Teachings on Cultivating Fearlessness and Compassion, by Pema Chodron

Fear: Essential Wisdom for Getting Through the Storm, by Thich Nhat Hanh

Love and Rage: The Path of Liberation Through Anger, by Lama Rod Owens

Radical Acceptance: Embracing Your Life with the Heart of a Buddha, by Tara Brach

Radical Compassion: Learning to Love Yourself and Your World with the Practice of RAIN, by Tara Brach

Soul Without Shame: A Guide to Liberating Yourself from the Judge Within, by Byron Brown

This Here Flesh: Spirituality, Liberation, and the Stories That Make Us, by Cole Arthur Riley

Trusting Change: Finding Our Way Through Personal and Global Transformation, by Karen Hering

When Things Fall Apart: Heart Advice for Difficult Times, by Pema Chodron

Other Online Resources

Self-Compassion Practices by Kristin Neff: self-compassion.org/self-compassion-practices

Creaky Joints, an international digital community of arthritis patients and caregivers: creakyjoints.org

The Nap Ministry: thenapministry.wordpress.com

Insight Timer app. Offers hundreds of guided meditations and a simple meditation timer: insighttimer.com

Website of Buddhist teacher Tara Brach, with guided meditations and talks: tarabrach.com

Cloud Way Website of Zenshin Florence Caplow, with links to teachings and classes: cloudway.live